Ten Ways to Straight A's

The Complete Guide to Success in School and Beyond

Sorelle Merkur

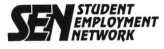

STUDENT
EMPLOYMENT
NETWORK

Toronto, Ontario

Published By:

Student Employment Network
117 Gerrard Street East, Suite 1002
Toronto, Ontario
M5B 2L4
Tel: (416) 971-5090
Fax: (416) 977-3782
E-mail: sen@studentjobs.com
Internet: http://www.studentjobs.com

Kevin E. Makra, Publisher/Editor

Cover Design: Matt Labutte

Editor: Douglas Duke

Tri-Graphic Printing (Ottawa) Limited

Printed in Canada

Canadian Cataloguing in Publication (CIP):

Merkur, Sorelle, 1978-
   Ten ways to straight A's : a complete guide to success in school and beyond

Includes index.
ISBN 1-896324-36-3

1. Study Skills
I. Student Employment Network (Toronto, Ont.).
II. Title.

LB2395.M47 2000   378.1'70281   C00-932596-4

ACKNOWLEDGMENTS

I would like to acknowledge the following people for helping me in the creation of this book: My mother, for dedicating her time, energy, and effort (not to mention support) to help me write and edit this book from start to finish; my father, for teaching me all that I know about school success and beyond; my older brothers, for pushing me to outdo their own accomplishments; Matt, for not only giving me the love that I needed to write this book, but also for motivating me to start writing this book in the first place and continuing to support me right until the end of it; my friends, who graciously accepted my work habits during the summer that I finished this book; those professors and teachers throughout my education who believed in my abilities and motivated me to strive for success; Barbara Simmons, for her efforts in making this book possible. Finally, I'd like to acknowledge my publisher who gave me the reassurance and support that I needed to write my first book. And, my editor, who helped me find the words to express all that I was trying to say.

TABLE OF CONTENTS

INTRODUCTION

How I Came To Write This Book

"I give up! I can't do this!" I mumbled to Gail, the woman who taught the art classes I took the summer before heading off to law school. I was talking about a painting that I was trying to copy – I just couldn't get it to look right. As I sat there frustrated by my inability to do what seemed to be a relatively simple task, the idea to write this book emerged. Now, you're probably wondering how I can possibly connect my frustration in an art class to a book about getting A's in university. Well, I promise you it will all make sense if you just keep reading.

"So, the economics student's having trouble painting, is she?" my art teacher teased. "It couldn't possibly be as difficult as getting into Harvard, could it?"

Then I started to think about what she said. I'm certainly no genius. Nor am I a bookworm, a nerd, or a browner. However, I *did* get into Harvard Law School. But it really wasn't as difficult as my art teacher was making it out to be. I'm truly convinced that pretty well anybody could get into an Ivy League school if they just had the right approach.

"Actually," I explained to her, "getting into Harvard isn't half as hard as painting this picture." Just in case you're as confused by this comment as my art teacher seemed to be, I'll explain what I meant.

The truth is, the people who do well in school are not necessarily the most intelligent or the most hardworking. There are a lot of geniuses out there who will never be at the top of their class – I know a fair share of them myself! And there are probably even more people who spend most of their waking hours immersed in schoolwork and still don't get the grades they're hoping for. Those who do excel in school aren't really any smarter than the average student. So what do they have, if not ability? Quite simply, they know *how* to do well. They've learned *'the system'*. I've created my own system for getting straight A's and I'm about to share it with you.

What Is This Book About?

School success opens the door to many opportunities. An excellent transcript can get you the job interview you've been hoping for your whole life. It can also get you into the graduate program of your dreams (as it did in my case). So, making your mark in school can put you in the best position for your future, whatever it may be.

But, how do you achieve school success? I'll tell you all about my personal system for success in this book. I've developed, perfected, and promoted this system throughout my years in high school and university. Within the ten chapters of this book, you will get to know the *10 Ways to Straight A's*. The best part is, it's simple!

If you read this book, you will learn how to get the most out of being in class, what to do to prepare for class, how to study for exams, and how to write effective papers. I will guide you through a step-by-step game plan for school success. Inevitably, reading this book will save you the time and energy it would have taken to develop a successful system on your own by trial and error.

Who Should Read This Book?

Are you currently a student, or are you soon to become one? Or are you thinking about going back to school? If so, this book is a must for you. The earlier you read this book, the better. Any delay in reading this book and you'll be forced to unlearn your bad study habits later on. Read it as soon as possible for the best results.

While this book tends to focus on university and college, I have made sure that it is applicable to all students, as early as Junior High School and as late as post-graduate studies. I present a method of school success that works, regardless of your current level of education.

I also want to make it clear that I use the terms 'university' and 'college' interchangeably in this book. I understand that the term 'college' means something different in the United States than it does in Canada but let's not get caught up with terminology. Rather, focus on learning the techniques that I present for succeeding in school. Most of them will apply to you regardless of where you are in your education at the present time.

What Makes This Book Different?

This book is different from any other book you've read on how to achieve school success and I'll tell you why. Frankly, I have a different theory about why some people succeed in school while others don't. I truly believe that nearly anyone can do very well academically. It's just a question of knowing what to do and then being committed to doing it. It's certainly not about how smart you are nor does it have anything to do with your past academic record.

After one of my brothers read over the first chapter of my book, he challenged me. "Now, wait a minute," he said. "Are you trying to say that anyone can get an 'A' or be at the top of his or her class? How do you define success, anyway?" We debated about whether people should set 'realistic' goals (i.e. aim to do a little better than the previous year) or whether they should just aim for 'success' in the general sense of the word.

I reminded my older brother that, ever since I was little, he had teased me that I was stupid. You see, as a little kid I never could calculate math problems in my head the way he could, I wasn't a fast reader, and I never pronounced words properly when I read them aloud. In general, I just didn't seem like a very bright kid. Perhaps the repetition of him calling me "stupid" really stuck in my head over the years and left me with a bit of a complex. Perhaps I really believed I was as stupid as he'd been telling me all my life.

Fortunately, this complex only served to help me. How? Well first, it made me realize at a fairly early age that I wasn't going to succeed in school on my brainpower alone. I had to find a creative way to achieve school success. So, what I set out to do was develop a foolproof system for doing well. I have stuck to this system throughout my high school and undergraduate years and will continue with it into the next stage of my education. My system has been instrumental in helping me achieve high marks, which in turn, has led to my winning numerous scholarships and awards that have financed my university education. Now, this system has landed me at one of the most prestigious law schools in the world (with a fellowship to help pay for it).

Who knows what would have happened had I set more "realistic goals". I doubt that I would have been where I am today. I believe people have to stop thinking about their limitations and start thinking about their possibilities. If you want to really achieve, you need to **think big**! That is, you've got to realize that there is nothing keeping you from making your mark in school, however big you'd like that mark to be. All you really need is some know-how. That's what I'm going to share with you.

In this book, I provide you with the tools that you'll need. It's all pretty straightforward. If you follow my system for achieving school success, you should have no problem achieving your goals. So, set your goals high and hold on tight.

How To Learn The 10 Ways To A's

Each chapter in this book presents a separate step in achieving school success. I'll take you through each step slowly and carefully to make sure that you fully understand what I'm trying to say. To help these lessons really sink in, I'll highlight important points throughout each chapter. I'll also include various exercises to get you involved along the way.

The best thing you can do is sit back and immerse yourself in this book. It's easy to read, and after you've put it down, you'll be surprised at how much you've learned in such a short period of time. Pretty soon, you'll notice that you're becoming a more organized and focused individual who knows how to do well.

25 Skills You Will Acquire From Reading This Book

If you follow my suggestions, you'll develop the skills to achieve school success:

1. Setting your goals for school success – and setting them early.

2. Prioritizing your activities and responsibilities at school.

3. Determining where academic success fits into your priorities.

4. Letting go of misconceptions that will only constrict the way you think.

5. Choosing your classes before heading off to school.

6. Deciding where to live while at school.

7. Financing your education (by looking for jobs, getting financial aid, or applying for scholarships).

8. Always attending classes and tutorials.

9. Preparing yourself properly before you go to class.

10. Taking complete and accurate class notes.

11. Using a method for taking thorough notes from textbooks and articles.

12. Keeping yourself organized during the school year.

13. Completing assignments and exercises correctly.

14. Forming positive relationships with classmates, older students, and professors.

15. Getting the best reference letters possible from your professors.

16. Preparing your notes and getting them ready for exam time.

17. Creating a schedule for yourself (using the *Wrap Around Scheduling System*) to keep you on target during exam time.

18. Using past exams to supplement your studying.

19. Finding a study method and sticking to it (the ICE Method: Issue Condensation Method for Exams).

20. Writing multiple-choice, open book, take home, and essay exams.

21. Surviving exam time by keeping calm, getting into a routine, and finding a good place to study.

22. Writing excellent papers and essays.

23. Using a method to essay writing that includes choosing a topic, doing the research, writing the paper, and editing it.

24. Learning how to avoid plagiarizing by footnoting properly and consistently.

25. Having a life at school by being well-rounded, taking care of yourself, and putting things in perspective.

Overview Of This Book

Each chapter of the book discusses one of my *10 Ways to Straight A's.* In each chapter, I lead you step-by-step through the process of achieving school success.

Chapter One: Shows you how to get your mind set on school success by setting your goals, prioritizing, and doing away with preconceived ideas that will only constrict the way you think.

Chapter Two: Teaches you how to prepare yourself before you head off to school. You've got to choose your classes, decide where to live, and determine how you will finance your education.

Chapter Three: Instills in you the importance of going to class and tutorials, and teaches you how to prepare for them.

Chapter Four: Leads you through the process of taking notes in class, from textbooks, and from articles that you are assigned.

Chapter Five: Discusses the importance of networking. You've got to know how to form positive relationships with your classmates, older students, professors and teaching assistants/fellows.

Chapter Six: This chapter will help you organize yourself for exam time. You need to prepare your notes, make a schedule using the *Wrap-Around Scheduling System*, and obtain resources such as past exams to study from.

Chapter Seven: You've got to use a study method for exams. I'll teach you about my own study method, the ICE Method (Issue Condensation for

Exam Method). It works, it's efficient, and you can use it to study for almost all of your courses.

Chapter Eight: I'll show you how to get through exam time with your nerves intact. I'll give you tips on how to keep calm, get into a routine, and find a comfortable place to study.

Chapter Nine: In this chapter I give you a step-by-step process for writing excellent papers and essays that includes choosing your topic, doing the research, writing the paper, and finally, editing it.

Chapter Ten: Success goes beyond school. You've really got to balance life while you're at school. You do this by being well-rounded, taking care of yourself, and putting things in perspective.

Follow the *10 Ways to Straight A's* and you'll breeze through achieving the school success you desire.

CHAPTER 1

GET YOUR MIND SET ON SCHOOL SUCCESS

Have you ever run a marathon, gone on a treacherous bike ride, or given a challenging stage performance? If so, I'm sure you quickly discovered the benefits of maintaining a positive attitude. Succeeding in school can be a similar experience. Doing well in university requires, first and foremost, a mind that is set on success.

In this chapter, I take you through three steps that will get you to think like a straight 'A' student. The **first step** is setting your goals. Deciding right away that you want to be successful in school will make achieving success easier and much more likely. Prioritizing is the **second step**. To achieve success in university or college, you must make school one of your top priorities. The **third step**, and perhaps most important step towards getting your mind set on success, is to get rid of any negative ideas you have about university or your own capabilities. If you take my advice and follow these three suggestions, you will certainly be in the right mind-set to make your mark at school.

Set Your Goals

Once you know what you want, it becomes much simpler to go after that goal and attain it. It's the same idea with school – you've got to set your goals and then tackle them head on.

Decide How Successful You Want To Be In School

When you enter your first year at college, you may already have plans for your future, like going into medicine, law, teaching, or whatever else may appeal to you. However, most of you, like myself, will find that three or four years of school can significantly change your idea of the kind of career you want or the type of career that would best suit you. There can be many unpredictable turns in the road you take. So, instead of concentrating on specific career goals, it would be a far more useful tactic to decide *how successful you want to be in school.* Then, when the time finally comes to make decisions about your future beyond university, you will have more opportunities available to choose from.

All of the self-help books out there (or at least the ones I've read) emphasize: "Successful people set goals!" While I agree that this has become something of an annoying cliché, I have to admit that it does have a lot of truth to it. If you do end up succeeding at something, then you probably started out with a clear intention to do just that. The same principle applies to succeeding in school.

Now I'm not implying that you should gather your family together and tell them that you plan on becoming President. And it may not be realistic to assume you'll be the next Bill Gates. But, if you do want to succeed at school, simply make that decision from the start. Setting a goal as early as possible will make achieving that goal so much easier.

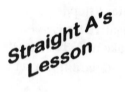 Instead of focusing on specific career goals, make school success your number one goal.

A Personal Anecdote

When I was deciding which university I should attend, my choices were narrowed down to Cornell University in Ithaca, New York and McGill University in Montreal, Canada. Ultimately, given the fact that there were significant differences in the tuition fees of the two schools, the decision became a financial one and I opted for McGill. However, as I left for Montreal, my parents promised me that if I ever had the opportunity to go to an Ivy League school for a graduate program, they would help me pay the tuition. So, as I began McGill, I was motivated to be accepted after undergrad into an Ivy League graduate program. I am now taking my parents up on their long-forgotten promise and I am currently attending Harvard Law School. So, you must never underestimate the importance of having goals. Without them, you might not always be able to justify why you're working so hard. However, if you have a clear focus, you can easily answer that question and reassure yourself that you are not wasting your time.

By the way, I'm not suggesting that you should set your goal on Harvard. But even if there is just a small part of you that is itching to make your mark, the best time to acknowledge that ambition is now. If you really do want to succeed, you can! I am going to tell you how to do it. Attaining success in school is simple: You need a practical guide and a willingness to work hard. In this book I have outlined a thorough and foolproof formula. Just stick to the *10 Ways to Straight A's*! By setting goals for yourself, you are taking the first step.

Straight A's Lesson   **If you have a clear goal to succeed, you won't feel that you're wasting your time working hard in school.**

Set Your Goals Early (But don't give up if your first year was a mess, there's still room for success)

The momentum for success gets launched in your very first year at college or university. However, if you do screw up in first year, as many people do, realize that you can get back on track the following year if you follow my suggestions. Don't give up, whatever you do!

At the same time, keep in mind that the grades you earn in your first year are just as important as those in any other year. Therefore, it really is best to start a reliable trend that can be maintained throughout your university career. Set your goals early and decide whether or not you really want to excel. If you do make the commitment to excel, this book can help you accomplish your goals.

Straight A's Lesson   **Decide you want to succeed early on. First year counts just as much as any other year so don't delay in setting your goals.**

Exercise

Get Yourself Psyched Up For School Success

Simply sitting back casually, holding this book with one hand while your other hand flips through the channels on your television, isn't going to help you in setting your goals. You've got to take goal setting seriously to reap the benefits. Here are some suggestions that will help get you psyched up with goals for school success:

Visualization: My mother, a therapist, has always taught me to picture myself succeeding at something in order for it to become a reality. Why don't you try this out for yourself! Imagine yourself at the end of your university or college program, walking up to receive your diploma while your list of awards and distinctions are being recited over the microphone. Amplify the scene by visualizing what you're wearing and who's there alongside you. Notice how satisfying it feels inside of you to be placed in that situation.

Write a list: Sit down with a large pad of paper and simply try to create a list of your goals in school. If that means simply writing out "I want to succeed!" over and over again, then do it!

Write a letter to yourself: Pretend you've just finished school. Try to imagine how you would feel if you really did accomplish your academic goals. Then, write a letter to yourself as you are right now, conveying the feelings of accomplishment and satisfaction that you imagine.

Prioritize

You've set your academic goals for college, but you can't help feeling that there are a lot of other things in your life that you care about besides school. It's time to start *prioritizing*.

Know What's Important To You

If someone came up to you out of the blue and asked you what you felt was the most important thing in your life, you might quickly answer, "My new car, of course." Perhaps that really might have been the first thing that came to your mind. However, if you were given time to really think about this question, I wonder what your answer might be then. University is a practical time to start thinking along such lines. Because there are so many things that tug at your time in university, it is helpful to personally assess what are the more important – and less important – things in your life. That way, you'll be able to rest assured that you are putting more time and energy into the activities you value most.

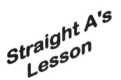

Decide what is important to you in university so that you can put your energy in the right places. Now is a good time to write down your own list of priorities.

Put Your Priorities In Order

Now that you've figured out what's important to you (or you've at least made your best guess), it's time to put those priorities into some sort of order. Your list is likely made up of some of the following things (these are not in any particular order):

family
friends
pet
boyfriend/girlfriend
exercise/sports
television/video games
school
fraternity/sorority
extracurricular activities (i.e. school newspaper, student council)
volunteer work/job
religion
other

Now that you have a list of the most important things in your life, it's time to put them in order of their actual importance to you. Understand that this exercise is only for your benefit. No one is judging your list, so be truthful.

1. _____
2. _____
3. _____
4. _____
5. _____
6. _____
7. _____
8. _____
9. _____
10. _____
11. _____
12. _____

Determine Where Academic Success Fits Into Your Priorities

Now I have a slightly different twist to this exercise: Arrange the same list in the order of what you think your priorities *should* be. This is where the concept of *priority* really comes into play. For example, you may like hanging out with your friends more than you like the idea of spending Sunday in the library. However, now you must decide which of those two activities *should* be more important to you.

1. _____
2. _____
3. _____
4. _____
5. _____
6. _____
7. _____
8. _____
9. _____

10. _____
11. _____
12. _____

If you really want to do well in school, it's likely that you placed school in one of the top three positions. And, to be honest, in order to be truly successful in university, school does need to be one of your top priorities. The truth is, you're going to have to make some sacrifices. In other words, you have to *prioritize* to accomplish your academic goals.

This second list isn't just a fantasy. Don't think: "Okay, I put school first or second, but I know that once it comes down to a choice between studying for an English exam or watching *Friends*, I'm going to choose *Friends* every time." Instead, stick to your ideal priority list and actually put school ahead of the Thursday night 'Must See TV' schedule. Even if your life does seem to revolve around a TV show, you can always tape it and watch it *after your exam is over.*

Don't worry if in the past you haven't made school a top priority. University, as I will discuss in the next section, wipes the slate clean. Whatever happened before is history; you can start again. It's not too late to rearrange your priorities!

This is not to say that you have to neglect other aspects of your life in order to succeed in school. Realistically, you might need to maintain a part-time job to get yourself through school, or you might be attending school on an athletic scholarship. Your priorities will obviously change depending on the situation you're in. Nevertheless, the higher up school is on your priority list, the more likely you'll be dedicated to doing well at it.

Straight A's Lesson

The people who do well in school usually place school as one of their top priorities even if it means making some sacrifices.

Do Away With Preconceived Ideas

University is a brand new chapter in your life and you should treat it that way. You've probably come to school with a lot of preconceived notions. These ideas might lead you to form quick but not necessarily helpful opinions. For example, you might already have formed an idea of yourself from high school that is less than admirable. Whatever these preconceptions might be, try to forget about them since they will only constrict your way of thinking. Keep your mind open to new ideas, new experiences, and new positive visions of yourself. After all, university is really about enlarging and challenging your perspective.

See Yourself As Successful

Whatever happened in high school – forget it! Whatever you think you can or cannot accomplish – don't worry about it! One of the wonderful things about university is that no records come with you. Even if you failed the twelfth grade miserably and you managed to get into university only because the admissions office made a mistake – who cares? Certainly not your professors or your classmates since they're unaware of your past failures and successes.

When you enter university or college, your grade point average is non-existent and your reputation is unblemished. So take this new beginning and make the most of it. There are no limits to what you can accomplish now. When you apply to graduate programs or to a job at the end of school, the only grades that will count will be the ones you've been piling up during your undergraduate years.

I'll say it again: University is a clean slate! Promise yourself right now to leave behind any negative ideas you may have formed about yourself. Instead, think of yourself now as a person who is successful. That visualization will give you the boost that you need to succeed.

Straight A's Lesson

Don't be constrained by any preconceived notions that you may have of yourself. Decide that you will be successful at college, and, as long as you follow the advice given in this book, you definitely will be.

Don't Believe The Misconception Of The Successful Student

Misconception: Successful people have no friends. They spend every single day and night at the library. They never go out. They wear pants that are way too short. They always sit in the same seat in the front row of the class, and come a half an hour early to get it. They run up to the professor after every lecture to carry the professor's books. They are *nerds*, *browners*, and *losers!*

If this truly were an accurate description of every successful student in college, then I might not blame you for choosing not to succeed. Who knows, perhaps you do know one or two people who fit this description and who are really successful. My point here is that if you think there is a singular profile of a successful student, you couldn't be more wrong. You can't spot successful people by their dress, nor can you pick them out based on where they sit in class. It's time to drop this misconception.

You can be a successful student without having to change the way you look. You can still have friends and you can even go out and have a good time. Being successful doesn't mean you have to devote every waking minute to studying. Balancing your work with time for yourself to do whatever you choose actually benefits your work and helps you achieve success. Do away with the misconception that schoolwork must take over your whole life in order to become a successful student. Being successful requires a *system* of doing well, but it doesn't require you to give up everything else in your life.

Straight A's Lesson

Don't think that to become successful, schoolwork must overtake your life. If you have a system of doing well in college, you can definitely do well and still have a good time.

Forget About These Three Other Misconceptions

Misconception 1: All professors are out to get you.

Don't allow yourself to form the attitude that professors are evil beings and just want to make your life as a student miserable. In fact, most professors want nothing more than to see their students do well and are happy to help them along in any way they can. Developing the attitude that professors really are on your side will make success seem so much more attainable. Professors are human. That means that they go through divorces, breakups, losses, and they also get sick once in a while. So, on the off chance that you approach a professor, and he/she treats you like you just killed their dog, don't run away and hide in your dorm room for the rest of the semester. Instead, assume that someone *else* killed the dog and you just caught your professor at a bad moment.

Misconception 2: There's just an impossible amount of work to do.

Your older brothers and sisters, or friends of the family, might successfully scare you before you get to university. They might paint you a picture, describing a life of endless reading, an infinite amount of assignments, and lectures that drag on forever. Initially, you might feel that their descriptions are accurate. However, as a recent graduate, I guarantee that in most classes, with a little hard work and a clearly constructed game plan, you can finish all the work and learn it well. Certainly, the amount of work is not infinite. Just don't give up right at the beginning simply because you have this misconception. Stick it out and you'll see that you too can get through it.

Misconception 3: There are easy courses; there are impossible courses.

"You have to take this course, it's an easy A … You can't take that course, I know the professor, and he's impossible!" Information like this is always good to know. However, be wary! There simply is no such thing as a course that will *guarantee* you an excellent mark. Likewise, no class is completely impossible to conquer. Generally, courses fall somewhere in the middle range of difficulty. Don't be intimidated by all of the standard myths. In the end, you'll discover how much you have to work in each of your courses to get the grades you're aiming for.

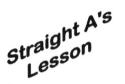

Forget your preconceived ideas about vindictive professors, an infinite amount of work, and impossible courses. Don't agonize over these ideas since most are merely exaggerations and misconceptions.

Summary

You're on your way to achieving straight A's by getting into the right mind-set, a mind-set that says, "I'm definitely going to do well this year!" After reading this chapter, you should realize that in order to succeed in school, you have to decide that you want to succeed, set your priorities accordingly, and forget about any misinformed ideas you may have developed.

CHAPTER 2

PREPARE YOURSELF BEFORE YOU HEAD OFF TO SCHOOL

"I'm leaving for school in three days, and I still haven't chosen my courses, I still haven't found a place to live, and I still don't know how I'm paying for everything!"

I wouldn't want to be in this person's shoes and I'm sure you wouldn't want to either. No doubt there are a lot of decisions to be made before you even step on to the university campus. Decisions that have to do with your classes, your living conditions, and your financial situation are very important and will have a significant impact on your success. Since they contribute greatly to shaping your school experience, you should consider each of these decisions very carefully. Getting your year off to a smooth start will allow you to stay relaxed and to concentrate on what's important to you.

Choose Your Classes

After weeks and weeks of you stalking the postal carrier, 'the letter' finally arrives. You got into the school of your dreams! You're ecstatic! All too soon though you come down from Cloud Nine when you realize you have to choose your courses for your first year at college. You'll have to go through the requisite questions and advice from your parents or older brothers and sisters such as, "You should take a computer class. That could be very useful when you're looking for a job," or "Aren't you at least going to *try* a business class?" Once all that is out of the way, you can sit down at your kitchen table – just you and that enormous student handbook you were sent by administration – and choose your classes for your first year at school. In no time you might feel a full-out panic attack coming on - you realize you don't have a clue where to begin.

Here are some important tips that will help you when you are mapping out your schedule:

Choose Classes That Interest You

First of all, make sure that you are interested in the classes you choose. It's easy to copy a friend's schedule – the prospect of being in class with someone you know is comforting – but this doesn't always work out. Your friend could drop the class and you'd be left stuck in a course that you were only taking because of someone who isn't even around anymore. Or, you may decide on a course because of its reputation for being a "bird course" (i.e. an extremely easy course). Don't rely too much on this myth. You'll still have to go to class, and you'll still need to study. And if the class is so seemingly insignificant that no one ever shows up to it, then come exam time studying will seem more difficult than you ever imagined. Other, more practical types of people, may decide to take classes according to the days of the week the classes are scheduled (this was my own personal favorite). But if you choose your courses according to this method, you'll end up wasting time in classes that you really don't care about.

If you have a genuine interest in a class, studying for it will be a lot less difficult because you won't feel that you're wasting your time. Also, keep in mind that if you take classes that interest you, you'll be more likely to end up in a career that will also interest you. Determine what you like and then go for it.

In order to choose classes you're interested in, you have to determine what subjects stimulate you. This is more difficult than it seems. When you're good at something, you might assume – as I often did – that it means you must like it. Typically, people find those things that come easy to them to be more enjoyable. Having an interest in something, and, at the same time, being good at it, is a win-win situation. But, convincing yourself that you have an interest in something just because you are good at it is not the same thing at all. Be careful when you choose your classes! Assess what you like and not simply what you're good at.

An important side-note here is that university is not only about finding out what kind of career you want and taking every single course in that particular area. The advantage of a liberal arts education is that it allows you to sample a variety of courses that might be totally unrelated to the one you are majoring in. So take advantage of this. If you do, you will probably leave university not only a successful academic but also an interesting person.

Straight A's Lesson

Take classes that interest you. If you are interested in a class, studying for it will be that much easier. As a result, doing well will come with much less of a struggle.

Do Research Before Signing Up For Courses

A second important piece of advice: Don't blindly sign up for classes – research them first! Whatever courses you do choose, remember that you'll be stuck in them for at least a semester and possibly a full year. So, don't make your decisions lightly as though you're ordering dinner at a drive-through restaurant. Spend some time actually looking into classes before you commit yourself to them.

Here is a checklist of what you should be finding out about your prospective classes:

1. The general material that will be covered in the course.
2. Who the professor is and what he/she is like, including teaching style.
3. The level of difficulty of the class.
4. Breakdown of the class marking-scheme (e.g. If there is no midterm and no essay, the final exam will be worth one hundred percent. If that prospect makes your hair stand on end, strike it off your list).
5. Time, date, and place of the class (If you schedule two classes side by side that are on completely opposite sides of campus, you might end up missing a significant part of each lecture).

So, how do you get this information? Here are a few suggestions:

1. **Older students**: Students a few years ahead of you in school, who you trust, and, who seem to have similar interests to you, can be a helpful source of advice when choosing your classes.

2. **Internet**: Go to your school's home page and then search for the class you're researching. There may be an outline of the course posted. If not, you can get the professor's e-mail address from the website and e-mail her/him for more information. As long as you

start your information search early, you'll give your professor enough time to respond to your queries before you have to finally decide.

3. **Advisors**: Advisors are always available to help you build a class schedule. They have detailed knowledge of the required courses for your particular program. So don't forget about them if you're having problems. You probably don't even have to show up at their office. There are almost always counselors/advisors at universities who will respond to your e-mails with detailed advice.

4. **Class evaluations**: Look at professor and class evaluations that are probably on reserve at your library. These ratings and comments might give you a good idea of what to expect in the course since other students from previous years wrote them.

5. **Bookstore**: Go to your school's bookstore to look at the textbooks assigned for different classes. See if you're drawn to them.

6. **Student handbook**: The description of classes is usually fairly accurate in these handbooks.

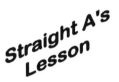

Do research before you commit yourself to a class for the year. Make the effort to contact people such as older students and school advisors to learn about the different courses you're considering. You want to find out about their difficulty levels, the professors teaching them, and the mark-breakdowns.

The benefits of looking into the classes you are signing up for may seem quite obvious, but its importance can't be stressed enough. If you ask the right questions and are persistent in looking into your courses, you will be less likely to be surprised in the middle of the year. This can be an important preventative measure to help you do well in school.

Create A Balance In Your Class Schedule

Choosing the right blend of courses each year is a balancing act in a lot of ways. Being able to do well in a course and taking courses that interest you are both important objectives when deciding what courses to take. However, it is important to create a balance between fulfilling these two objectives. A schedule that is filled with courses that are easy A's might make you happy because you have so much time to do everything else college has to offer. But, this situation is also unsatisfying because you did go to university to learn about something that interests you and that will prepare you for your future. At the same time, taking a course load full of intellectually challenging courses might make your hair fall out when you realize that having enough time for all of them will require skipping all your meals for the rest of the year.

Create a schedule that combines intellectually challenging classes with a few fun courses that are less time-consuming.

Exercise

Mapping Out Your Years In School

If you haven't done this yet, then it's a good idea to map out your years at university/college and the courses that you are planning to take. You want to ensure you'll have all the credits you need to graduate on time.

Talk to an advisor to make sure that:

1. You are fulfilling all the requirements for your degree or major.
2. You'll have completed any necessary prerequisites for your courses.
3. You're scheduled to finish your degree on time.
4. You are not taking too many out-of-faculty courses.
5. You'll have enough credits to graduate.
6. All your electives will count towards your degree.

Straight A's Lesson

Create a schedule that balances interesting intellectual courses with courses that are more relaxing and less time consuming.

Decide Where To Live

Whatever year of university you are entering, you'll have to decide where you should live. This decision can come back to haunt you if you end up choosing a roommate or an apartment that you don't like. Living in a place that's peaceful and comfortable will make it a lot easier to concentrate on getting the grades you want. So, be sure to make this decision carefully.

Dorms vs. Apartments

If you haven't yet decided whether to live in a dorm or an apartment, let me give you some insight into both situations. There are definitely pros and cons to living in each type of environment that you should understand before you commit yourself to either one.

The Advantages Of Dorms:

1. More social.
2. Usually less expensive than maintaining your own apartment.
3. No bills to worry about.
4. Easier to maintain (i.e. Dorm rooms are usually smaller so they are easier to keep clean and bathrooms are usually cleaned by staff).
5. No need to buy furniture.
6. No food preparation or food shopping.
7. Most dorms are close to campus whereas a lot of apartments are far away.
8. You can always find someone around to help you out whether it's about a class or your personal life.

The Advantages Of Apartments:

1. More spacious.
2. Usually a lot quieter than dorms.

3. More control over the food you eat.
4. Amenities such as your own television, kitchen, and washroom.
5. Tend to have more privacy in an apartment than in a dorm room.
6. More control over the people you live with.

After you ponder the pros and cons of living in a dorm, you should be able to decide what's right for you. If you still aren't sure however, I suggest that living in a dorm room is a really good way to integrate yourself into school life in your first year. You meet a lot of people (people who are just as eager to meet you as you are to meet them), you learn the ropes from floor fellows/hall officers/resident assistants, and you get a chance to be independent without having to take on the full responsibility of keeping up an apartment. Living in a dorm can be a great way to spend your first year, and, by the time you become sick of it, you'll be ready and willing to move into an apartment for the next few years.

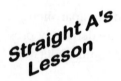

Straight A's Lesson

Living in a dorm is a good idea for your first year since it's an easy way to make you comfortable in your new surroundings at university.

Choosing A Dorm

A lot of people choose to live in dorms at some point in their university career. It's a great place to meet people and it's usually a lot simpler than keeping up an apartment. If you're one of the people who have decided to live in a dorm this year, then you're probably faced with a lot of decisions about which dorm to live in. Don't be too distraught over such a decision. Most dorms will be more than adequate and I'm sure you'll find friends and the kind of life you want wherever you end up. But, you still do have to make a decision so there are some things to think about.

Factors To Consider When Choosing A Dorm:

1. **Location**: If you want to be close to campus, eliminate all the dorms that you consider too far away. This will immediately make your decision simpler. How far the dorm is from the gym or the library may

be much more important to you than how far it is to class. So really think about where the dorm is located in relation to different places.

2. **Co-ed**: Some dorms at your university will be co-ed (they may all be) while others may not be. Think about which you prefer.

3. **Financial**: Some dorms may be more expensive than others. If your budget is tight (which for most students it is) then an easy way to save some money is by staying in the least expensive dorm.

4. **Multicultural**: Some dorms are housed predominantly by international students, but you can live there if you request it. If meeting students from around the world and opening your eyes to people from different nations would appeal to you, this could be the dorm for you.

5. **Noise Level**: At every educational institute, there are the dorms everyone knows as the "party dorms", and there are the dorms that are much more reserved. When you do choose a dorm, remember that being able to get a good night's sleep before a long day of classes or an exam might be difficult to do in a dorm with the 'party-all-night' reputation. You can always hang out there – but do you really want to live there?

6. **Bathrooms**: Being near a bathroom might be something you never really considered important. But if you have to walk down a long hall in the middle of the night to go to the bathroom you might be less than enthusiastic about your living quarters. You should know how many people in each dorm share a bathroom before you make your decision. In addition, bathrooms in some dorms might be co-ed (as they were at my university). I knew I would be uncomfortable sharing a bathroom with guys so I chose a dorm where the bathrooms weren't co-ed.

7. **Kitchens**: Some dorms will have a kitchen on every floor, some will have more than one, and some will have none. If you are a health nut or have an allergy to certain foods and you don't think you're going to find anything to eat in the cafeteria, try to stay in a dorm with at least one kitchen on your floor.

8. **Roommates**: Some dorms have single rooms while others often house two to a room. The thought of sharing a small room with someone you've never met might make you feel claustrophobic. On the other hand, the idea might be comforting to you. Your experience will differ greatly depending on whether you have a roommate or not. This is something important to consider.

9. **Study Rooms**: Often, dorms will be equipped with study rooms. These rooms are usually quiet and can be a nice change from the solitary confines of your own room.

Factors To Consider When Choosing A Floor And A Room In A Dorm:

1. **Quiet Floors**: If you're the kind of person who likes to work at home, or in your room, then you'll probably want to request a quiet floor.

2. **Smoking / Non-Smoking Floors**: If you're a non-smoker, make sure you indicate that and get a room on a non-smoking floor.

3. **Requesting A Friend**: If your best friend from high school is following you to university, you might really want to live next to him/her. On the other hand, you might want to surround yourself with people you didn't know in high school. The university often carries through on specific room requests so be careful what you request since you'll most likely get it.

4. **Requesting People In Your Program**: This is probably the smartest request you can make on your dorm card. Having people in your dorm that will be taking the same classes as you can be extremely helpful throughout the year. Some schools might even have specific dorms for different programs or faculties. If they do, you might want to consider requesting one of these.

5. **Special Needs**: If you have special needs, make sure that you get a note from your doctor highlighting these needs. For example, you can request a large room or request being on a low floor. Be truthful in your requests though, there are many people out there who do have special needs and there are only a limited number of spaces for them.

Whatever the case, you should be able to find a dorm, a floor, and a room, that suit your needs. However, you should also know that even if a dorm is known to be quiet, most of the time it will be difficult to get good work done in your room. Dorms, above anything else, are a social setting. As a result, you might find that the library becomes your best friend. When it comes time to really get serious about your work, you'll likely find that dorms are not the best place to study.

Straight A's Lesson

There are lots of things to think about when choosing a dorm, a floor, and a room in a dorm. Think about the factors that are important to you in a dorm such as its location, the noise level, and whether the dorm has single rooms or not. If you choose a dorm appropriately, you're more likely to be happy in the dorm and able to concentrate on doing well in school.

Choosing An Apartment

There are many more things to consider when choosing an apartment than when choosing a dorm. Still, a lot of the same factors apply.

Finding An Apartment: It can be more or less difficult depending on the city in which you are located.

Density of City: Some cities have so many students living in them that reasonable housing is very hard to find. Other cities are much more spread out and have a wide variety of housing to choose from.

Real Estate Agent: In some cities you can contact landlords directly to inquire about renting an apartment. In other cities, the protocol is that you find a real estate agent and get an apartment that way. The former is usually an easier and cheaper method because the latter method may require paying a "finder's fee" to the real estate agent. This fee could, for example, be the equivalent of one month's rent.

Finding an apartment these days has become so much easier with the use of the Internet. Most universities have their own site for apartment listings in the area. In addition, there are a number of useful Internet sites listed at the back of this book that can help you in your apartment search.

Factors To Consider When Finding/Renting An Apartment:

1. **Be Persistent**: The process of finding an apartment usually starts with an ad in the newspaper that has sparked your curiosity. This leads to a phone call where you inquire into the apartment's availability. If you are told that the apartment has already been rented, don't stop there. Ask whether the landlord has any other apartments available. After all, if the ad you read about in the paper sounded appealing, perhaps there are other similar apartments owned by the same landlord that are available.

2. **Price Range**: Before you even inquire about an available apartment, make sure you know what your price range is. You'll waste your time, a landlord's time, and a real estate agent's time if you haven't quite figured out how much you're willing to spend. You really want to be careful not to choose an apartment beyond your means since it would only create stress in your life and may force you to take on more part-time work than you were planning to.

3. **Location**: Where do you want to live? You might find that living a little further from campus can be cheaper in terms of rent. This might be something you want to think about if your finances are tight. However, living further away from campus might end up wasting too much of your time and might also become a problem if you have to walk home late at night by yourself.

4. **Safety**: This is probably the most important factor to consider for. Not feeling safe in your own apartment will make living there uncomfortable. If safety is a big concern for you, avoid living in places that are located in dark alleyways or are on the first floor of a building. In addition, windows should be secure and should not contain only a single pane of glass. There are most likely brochures at your university housing office outlining safety tips in the campus area. You might want to get your hands on one.

5. **Number of Bedrooms**: How big do you want your apartment to be? It obviously depends on the number of roommates you're planning to live

with. In the next section I discuss roommates and things to think about when choosing them.

6. **Noise Level**: Determine how loud you think your apartment is going to be. If you're the kind of person who likes to do your studying at home, this will be very important. First of all, if your apartment is on a main street it will probably be a lot noisier than if it is on a side street. Second of all, if there are a lot of fraternity and sorority houses in the area – often sites for many loud parties – you might want to rethink your options.

7. **Transportation**: If you are living far from campus and don't have a car, make sure there is some sort of public transportation available to get you to school.

8. **Pets**: Planning to have a pet with you while away at school may make finding an apartment a lot more difficult since a lot of apartments don't allow animals. You'll want to start your apartment search earlier than normal if you plan on bringing a pet to school.

9. **Lease Term**: Some landlords insist on leases longer than one year. Getting tied into a two-year lease can be very constricting and you probably should avoid it. On the other hand, you may get lucky and find a landlord who is willing to give you just an eight or nine month lease. This can be great since it allows you to avoid the summer rent, something particularly helpful in your last year.

10. **Utilities**: Utilities can be very expensive in many cities and especially so in ones that experience harsh winters. If your utilities are included in the rent, great! It makes budgeting your finances that much easier. If they aren't included however, it's not the end of the world. You should know exactly which utilities are and are not included in your rent (i.e. water, sewerage, hot water, heat, and electricity). Keep in mind that newer apartments tend to conserve heat more than older ones. Ask your landlord or the previous tenants of the apartment how much the utility bills averaged out to per month. When determining how much the apartment will cost you, be sure to include the projected utility bills.

11. **Laundry Facilities**: Unless you plan on wearing the same pair of underwear the entire year (and I hope for your classmates' sakes you're

not), then you had better make sure you'll have some way to do your laundry in your apartment building. If there are no laundry facilities, make sure that there is a coin laundry nearby or that you have made some arrangement to get your laundry done. Of course, there is always the option of renting a washer and dryer for the year, but it could get pretty expensive.

12. **Necessities**: In all your excitement, you may forget to check on some obvious necessities. Be certain that there is a working stove and refrigerator, and inquire as to whether or not there is a dishwasher, or a place for one in the kitchen, if need be.

13. **Amenities**: If you're the type of person who only feels at home in a place that's really comfortable, check out all of the amenities that are available in your apartment. Fireplaces, balconies, storage spaces, courtyards, carpets, etc. can only make your apartment living that much more enjoyable.

14. **Parking**: If you have a car, ask the landlord if parking is available in the building. Is it indoor or outdoor? Does it cost extra? If the building doesn't provide parking, be sure to find out if there is street parking or a garage nearby where you can rent a spot.

15. **Change Your Locks**: Insist that the locks to your front door be changed. You may know the person who is moving out of the apartment, but do you know who lived there before him/her?

16. **Signing A Lease**: The language on a lease is often confusing and arbitrary. Before you sign your lease, check whether the landlord has the power to raise your rent as the cost of living increases. Also, make sure that the figure you have agreed to pay as your rent is fixed for the duration of your lease. Don't sign clauses that allow the landlord to enter your apartment without you there, or without your explicit consent. This will avoid any quarrels should you find yourself dealing with an intrusive landlord.

Wherever you decide to live, make sure that it is comfortable, peaceful, and within your price range. That way, you'll be happy to return home at the end of your day. When you're happy with your home-life, it makes it that much easier to concentrate on your schoolwork.

Straight A's Lesson

Choose an apartment wisely by examining different factors such as the price, location and safety of the apartment. Make sure that it's conducive to a successful year at university.

Choosing A Roommate

When it comes to choosing a roommate, you've really got to know yourself, and the kind of person you will be compatible with in a living situation. Here are some points to consider:

- **Close Friends:** Just because someone's your closest friend doesn't mean you'll enjoy living with him/her. In fact, you might find that living together is the surest way to end a once amazing relationship. Think twice before you commit to living with your closest friend.

- **Cleanliness:** If you're sharing an apartment with someone, you're sharing all of your furniture and your space. There's definitely enough to keep you busy at university, so make sure the person you choose to live with knows how to keep a place relatively clean, otherwise you'll not only be a student, but also a housekeeper.

- **Selfishness:** Probably the worst quality in a roommate is selfishness. Although we all have selfish tendencies, living with a person who only thinks about himself/herself will drive you crazy. Imagine the night before an exam having to put up with a roommate blasting Pearl Jam at four o'clock in the morning!

- **Financial Compatibility:** You might know your friend inside and out. You know his/her favorite color, movie, television show, and album. However, it's unlikely you'll truly know that friend's financial situation. Sharing an apartment with someone makes financial responsibility very important. You've got to pay the rent, the bills, and take care of the apartment. Making sure your roommate is responsible in financial situations is difficult to find out but it is an important thing to consider. I suggest that before you commit to living with a roommate, you should discuss your budgets to see whether the two of you are financially compatible.

- **Mood Swings:** When you go out with your friends, you're all probably in a great mood. It's Friday night, you're going out partying, and none of you are worried about anything. Getting along in this situation is simple. However, it's a very different story when you live with people and you see them all the time. Then, you're not only seeing them when they're at their best, but you're also seeing them when they are studying, waking up, feeling sick, and experiencing all the other things that go on at university. As a result, people who tend to display huge mood swings might not be the best people to live with.

- **Communication:** No matter whom you live with, it's inevitable that you will face problems. Whatever these problems may be, you must be able talk about them with your roommate. Living with someone who cannot communicate his/her feelings and thoughts openly, honestly, and without undermining you will frustrate you enormously, so be prepared for it. If you do end up living with a poor communicator, set the example by being open about your own feelings.

No matter who you do decide to live with, it will all work out as long as you're willing to make the effort to solve any problems that may arise. Of course, being roommates shouldn't be all about problems and fights. Building a friendship out of a roommate situation will make school so much more enjoyable. You can also build a support system with your roommate right 'at home.' Being there for your roommate and letting your roommate be there for you will make your university experience much more rewarding.

Straight A's Lesson

Before choosing roommates, think about characteristics that are important for roommates to have, such as cleanliness, financial responsibility, and consideration for other people. Whoever you choose to live with, try to build a strong relationship with them. This will create a comforting support system for you at home.

Finance Your Education

With the rising cost of tuition each year, paying for school is becoming more and more of an issue. Figuring out your financial situation and then creating a budget for yourself is something that you must do before you start your school year. Keeping your financial situation under control is necessary to keep you sane. Not being able to buy groceries or pay your rent is a horrifying experience that you will want to avoid at all costs. In order to avoid these situations, you've got to be responsible right from the beginning. This requires three steps:

1. Figure out your total cost of living (including tuition, books, food, etc.) for the year.
2. Determine how much financing you need for the year.
3. Formulate a plan to finance your education.

Calculate Your Cost Of Attendance

The first thing you must do is figure out the total amount it will cost you to go to school for one year. (We'll refer to this as your total cost of attendance). This requires summing up all of the various expenses that you will incur during the school year. The student handbook from your university will give you a fairly accurate idea of what you should expect to spend on tuition, books, and health fees. The rest is up to you. I have made a work sheet for you to help you figure out your total cost of attendance.

Tuition:	_____
Books and Supplies:	_____
Health Fees:	_____
Room/Board:	_____
Personal:	_____
Food:	_____
Travel:	_____
Loan Fees:	_____
Total Cost of Attendance: (estimated)	_____

If you've done this exercise accurately, you can expect to spend close to your total cost of attendance over a year's time. This is as long as you stick to your budget and don't spend beyond your means.

Analyze Your Financial Situation

Now that you know the total cost of attendance for the year, you've got to determine what portion you'll be able to pay for, and the amount you will need from other sources to cover the remainder.

If your parents are able to pay for your university education, then obviously you won't have to worry much about this. What you will have to do is figure out how much money you will be getting from them each month and then calculate a monthly budget so that you don't end each month completely broke. Set a budget and stick to it!

If, for whatever reason, your parents are unable to help you out, then you have to take complete responsibility for the financing of your education. If you've worked for the past few summers then you probably have some savings in a bank account. Write down the amount that you can contribute to your education and subtract this amount from the total cost of attendance.

Total Cost of Attendance: _____

Your Personal Savings: - _____

Amount You're Short: _____

After this calculation, you should have an accurate idea of the amount of money that you'll need to come up with to be able to pay for university. It's time to look at ways to come up with that money.

Decide About Your Financing

There are many ways to pay for your university education, but robbing a bank is certainly not one of them! There is always the option of trying to get financial aid or applying for a loan. Your university will have all the information you need about both of these options (I have also listed many websites at the back of this book that will help you locate financial aid). I'm going to concentrate on the other ways to raise money for your education: Applying for scholarships or getting a summer or part-time job.

Scholarships

Whatever your financial situation is, scholarships can help out a great deal. Even if you're not in desperate need of the money, receiving a scholarship looks great on a resume. So really, there's no reason not to look into scholarship possibilities. There are many scholarships out there that people barely even know about. In fact, hundreds of thousands of dollars in untapped scholarship money is just sitting and waiting for your application to come along. All of these scholarships have different requirements attached to them - wouldn't it be great if you found the one that perfectly fits your qualifications? It would certainly alleviate some of the stress of paying for school.

But these scholarships won't just come to you on a silver platter. They take time to locate and even more time to apply for. However, these days the Internet is making scholarship searching so much easier.

Where To Find Out About Scholarships:

- **Your School:** The first place to start your scholarship search is in your high school guidance office when you're applying for college. There may be separate applications for scholarships that you may need to fill out for certain schools. If you've already attended a year or more at your university/college, go to the scholarship office at your school or locate its website to inquire about scholarship availability.

- **Religious Groups:** Many religious organizations and youth groups offer a great number of scholarships. If you are involved in any of these groups, make sure you ask a coordinator about scholarships.

- **Parents' Employers:** More and more companies offer scholarships to children of their employees.

- **Websites**: There are now hundreds of websites where you can search through scholarship databases for awards tailored to your needs and qualifications. I've listed some of the most comprehensive scholarship sites at the back of this book to get you on the right track.

Summer And Part-time Jobs

Getting a good summer job is a great idea for a number of reasons. Not only will it be an asset to your resume, but the money you earn will also help pay your bills during the school year. Spending your summer wisely is a super way to help finance your education.

You might find it difficult to get your dream summer job during your first and second year at college/university. Employers prefer candidates who are almost finished their degrees. Nevertheless, with a little effort you can definitely find excellent summer jobs where you can learn a great deal and get paid well. Even if you can't find a great job for your first or second summer of undergraduate studies, using a summer to volunteer at an organization or company will build up your resume and help you get a job the following year.

In my first year of undergrad studies I applied to dozens of summer jobs. Finally, I got a job working at the Royal Bank of Canada in their Summer Undergraduate Training Program. But, I had to apply to a lot of jobs to find just one. Persevere in your job search! Expect a lot of rejections and don't be disappointed when you get them. Continue your search until you find a satisfying offer and if you really can't find a summer job, then it's a good idea to consider volunteering to help build up your resume. With the experience you'll have gained, you'll be in a much better position to apply for jobs the following summer.

If you have to find a part-time job during the school year, be sure to start looking for one early. Having a job lined up for you before you go to school will be a lot less stressful than if you are forced to be searching for a job in your first three weeks of school. Even worse, a lot of employers get their staff lined up for the year during the summer. So, start your job search early in the summer if you are planning on having a part-time job during the school year.

Where To Find Summer And Part-time Jobs:

- **Your School**: The first place to look for job listings is your school's career services office. Throughout the year there will be listings of jobs and internships for the summer. Usually firms visit schools during the year to recruit students. Go to the information sessions held by these firms to find out about the specific characteristics the firms look for in an application and resume. The most important thing to do is to start your search early so you can make all of the deadlines for applying to these jobs. These deadlines can start as early as the end of October so don't delay in thinking about how you want to spend your summer.

- **Network**: When you are looking for a job, you want to tap into every possible resource at your disposal. If that means annoying your parents for phone numbers of their friends and relatives who work in places that might be hiring for the summer, then do it! Even if you know someone at a company who has nothing to do with hiring, just asking that person to put in a good word for you with the Human Resources department can make a huge difference. You've got to be aggressive in your job search and use all the resources you can to find a great job.

- **Websites**: There are hundreds of websites out there that post job listings. Use them in your job search. In addition, there are now a lot of jobs available on the Internet that you can do while sitting at home. This could be ideal for you as a student, since it would save travel time and let you create your own work schedule. There are tons of options out there so be comprehensive in your job search and find a job that suits your abilities and needs.

As long as you start early enough and put a lot of effort into your job search, you'll find something that suits your needs and abilities, and pays enough to contribute to the financing of your education.

Commonly Asked Questions

Question: What should I do about choosing a major?

Answer: While I didn't specifically address this question in this chapter, you should go about choosing a major in a similar way as you choose your classes. To refresh your memory, I emphasized the importance of choosing classes that interest you. Well, guess what? You should definitely choose a major that you find interesting. You'll be taking most of your classes in this field so you want to make sure that it stimulates you.

Choosing a major that you find easy (i.e. that you're able to do well in without working too hard) will definitely make your life a lot simpler. But, be careful not to choose a major simply because it's easy. If you're not interested in something – even if it comes naturally to you – you won't want to spend your time learning the material. And, you really don't want to end up in a career that isn't satisfying.

So, when choosing a major, decide what stimulates you the most and go for it.

Question: I have to maintain a part-time job while I'm in school. Do you think I can still get the grades I'm aiming for?

Answer: Definitely. In university, you've got to prioritize. One of your priorities will be to maintain a part-time job. As long as you make sure that school doesn't fall too far from the top of your priority list, you should still have enough time available for your studies. The method for school success that I present in this book centers on study efficiency. That is, you want to make the most out of every minute you spend studying. If you have a job cutting into your time, you'll probably be even more efficient when you're studying since you know you don't have any time to waste.

Summary

As you can see, there are a lot of decisions to be made before you head off to university – but don't worry! You've probably noticed these decisions don't require the knowledge of a rocket-scientist. With a little guidance and organization in advance, you can be well prepared. With your classes chosen, your living arrangements organized, and your finances all worked out, you'll be more than ready to settle down for a successful school year.

CHAPTER 3

GO TO CLASS PREPARED

If you've been a typical freshman, and chosen to watch *Days of Our Lives* over attending classes, then around exam time, you're probably going to be in the middle of a serious breakdown. Imagine a week before your big exam: You've been to a few classes (the days when your Soap was pre-empted, perhaps), you've done most of the readings, and you're feeling pretty good about your chances in next week's Poli-Sci exam. Then you start to flashback to your mother's warning, "You'd better go to class and not sit home all day watching TV." So, you start trying to hunt down lecture notes. Except you haven't been attending lectures and you don't know anyone else in the class. Then you hear about some kid who's a "friend of a friend" and he has lecture notes for about half the classes. You finally track him down, photocopy his notes and take them back to your dorm room to read only to discover you can't understand a thing because the guy has the handwriting of a four-year-old with bad penmanship.

What are your options now? At this point, there aren't many. You'll probably be stuck studying from what you learned from your textbook and a few articles, and perhaps from the one or two pages of lecture notes that you were able to decipher. This doesn't leave you in a very good position.

Most of the time, a textbook is only a *supplement* to the class lectures. If you haven't gone to class, you can't possibly write what the professor really wants to hear: His or her own words. Realizing early on that the key to school success is in attending classes will give you a real fighting chance to succeed. Without going to class, you've literally taken yourself out of the game before it's even begun.

You've got to go to class to get your A's. Do not forget that! By not attending lectures you make doing well infinitely more difficult. Now don't fret! I'm not going to repeat it to you over and over again: You have to go to class! You have to go to class! You have to go to class! Instead, in this chapter I'm going to give you several good reasons to attend classes regularly and to teach you how to prepare yourself properly for them. This chapter is probably the most important in the book because if you miss the point of going to class, you're never going to get the A's you're aiming for.

Go To Class

I'll tell you one final time: You've got to go to class to achieve school success. Let me explain to you some important reasons why this is the case. Whenever you forget why you're hauling yourself to school so early in the morning, think back to this section of the book to reassure yourself that going to class is not a waste of your time.

Classes Are Key To Determining What Course Material Is Most Important

You go into your first class and you're assigned a huge textbook and a reader full of articles. On top of it are all the lectures you must attend. After lugging everything back to your dorm room you sit back and say to yourself: "How am I ever going to read all this stuff and actually learn it?" After the first week of classes you come to the even more terrifying realization that each and every one of your classes have similar huge textbooks and readers.

Right about now, you see yourself with several possible choices:

a) Accept that it is totally impossible to do all the reading you've been assigned and quickly return everything to the bookstore for a full refund;

b) Start to panic and declare you're not leaving your dorm room until Christmas vacation; or

c) Decide to casually read through the readings during your favorite prime-time television shows.

In order to survive (and actually succeed) at university, you must be able to determine what is and is not important in each of your classes. Unfortunately, I myself didn't figure this out until my third year at university. Had I known it beforehand, my life would've been *a lot* easier *a lot* earlier! Let me relay to you the circumstances surrounding my epiphany.

After feeling the 'Junior blahs' at the beginning of my third year, I thought that it might be a nice change to enroll in a Film class. I decided to take Introduction to Film, a course that is usually reserved for first-year students. On the first day, my professor, Trevor Ponech, drew a Venn diagram to help us figure out what we should be concentrating on in terms of the lecture material, textbook reading, and articles that were assigned. The diagram looked like this:

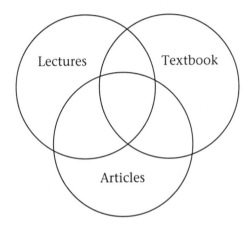

In many of your classes, you'll be assigned a textbook as well as several articles. On top of both of these are your class notes. The most important thing to learn is how to put all that material together and that's where the Venn diagram comes in. The area in which the textbook material, lecture material, and article material overlap should be your primary focus when studying. The professor knows it, I know it, and now I'm letting the whole world in on it.

What's my point? Simple: Missing classes is the single biggest waste of your time at university. Without attending your lectures, it's going to be impossible to determine what will definitely be on your exam, that is, the material in the intersection of your lecture material, textbook material, and article readings.

Predict Exam Questions

As long as you've attended your lectures on a regular basis, you should have a fairly good idea of what material is the most important to understand for an upcoming exam. As we've just gone over, it's that material where your lectures, your textbook readings, and your articles overlap. Now, let's find out how to put this valuable information to use.

As long as you know this information, it should be a breeze to fairly accurately predict the questions that will be on your exam. These 'predictable' questions will relate directly to the material that's centrally important to a course (i.e. that material that you've discussed in lecture and read about in articles and in your textbook).

Once you have the ability to accurately predict the questions that will be on an exam, you're way ahead of the game. Then, you can work on preparing your answers and learning them inside and out. Once you have formulated these questions, test yourself over and over to make sure that you'll be able to answer them perfectly. You're definitely going to feel like a prize student once you start accurately predicting questions and are able to give expertly prepared answers on an exam.

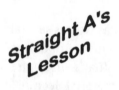

Attending lectures allows you to figure out what material is centrally important in a course. Using this information appropriately will help you predict questions that will appear on upcoming exams.

Professors And Their Egos

I've given you a diagram to emphasize how important it is to go to your classes – it's the key to figuring out what is and is not important for the exam. To drive this point home a little more, I'll put it to you even clearer. Lectures give your professor a forum to talk endlessly about a subject he or she is devoted to. An exam gives you a chance to show the professor you were paying attention during all of those lectures, out of respect and appreciation for his or her brilliance and expertise.

Professors have big egos! (I apologize if there are any professors out there reading this, but I have to tell what I feel is the truth!) They think they know a lot – and most of them do! And when they mark your exams, they will often give the highest marks to those students who echo their words. If you want to do well on an exam, you've got to know what the professor has said and be able to explain it back to him or her. Without going to class, this simply will not be possible.

Straight A's Lesson

To get a high mark on an exam, you've got to show the professor that you've been paying attention in your classes. You've got to go to class to be able to write a winning exam.

Even When You're Convinced A Class Is Useless – You Should Still Go

Let's say that you're taking a course where one large essay makes up one hundred percent of your final grade. The professor talks endlessly during lectures, but you know that that material will never show up on an exam because there just isn't going to be one. You could make a good case here that lectures are a little pointless.

Nevertheless, there still are reasons to continue to attend lectures besides the fact that you're paying a lot of money for the class and you should get the most out of it. The most important reason to keep attending lectures relates to the fact that professors tend to announce important deadlines and information during lecture time. Not knowing this important information can significantly hurt your grade. For example, the professor might during lecture announce that the deadline for your essay worth one hundred percent has been changed. Or, the professor may discuss the criteria that will be used to evaluate your essay or information he or she hopes you will include in your paper. There are a lot of comments and hints that the professor might occasionally spew out off the top of his or her head during these 'useless' lectures. You probably don't want to miss this information.

Straight A's Lesson

Even if you believe that the lectures in a course are completely useless, you should still go even if only to jot down important deadlines and other information that the professor conveys.

Go To Tutorials

In addition to lectures, many of your classes may also include tutorials. Typically, tutorials are small class-like sessions carried on with a teaching assistant or teaching fellow. You'll find that many students dismiss tutorials right away as being "a complete waste of time". However, if you give tutorials a chance, you'll realize that they really can be worthwhile.

My advice here is to consider tutorials part of your class. Go to your tutorials as consistently as you go to your classes. In this section I'll give you some important reasons to help you understand why you should make sure you attend your tutorials.

An Opportunity For Personal Attention

Because of their smaller size, tutorials are a good place to get the kind of one-on-one attention that regular classes lack. There, you can get answers to your and your classmates' questions. As well, tutorials are a great place to get a grasp on material that may have gone over your head in class (this is especially advantageous in science or math classes). The teaching assistant will likely discuss more complicated material at a much slower pace than that which the lecture offered. Attending tutorials can also save you the time it might otherwise have taken to schedule appointments with your professor during his or her office hours for help or advice. Generally, having a smaller session with a teaching assistant will help you learn the course material much more thoroughly.

Straight A's Lesson

Because tutorials are smaller than lectures, they give you the opportunity to ask questions and have them answered at a slower than normal pace.

Material Covered In Tutorials May Be On Your Exam

Even though your professor is not usually present at tutorial sessions, the material covered by the teaching assistant during them is almost always subject for examinations (unless otherwise specified). Your teaching assistant might discuss something in a tutorial that you've never examined in a lecture. This could be information that you need to know for an upcoming exam. Therefore, missing your tutorials is akin to missing your classes. The material covered in tutorials can be just as important and test-worthy as the material that your professor discusses in lecture.

Straight A's Lesson

Material that is covered in tutorials is often tested on exams even though it may not have been overtly discussed in a lecture.

Teaching Assistants/Fellows: The Hidden Gem

It might take you too long to realize this important piece of information, so I want to emphasize it now: Teaching assistants or teaching fellows often have more control over your mark in a course than your professors do. In a lot of courses, the teaching assistant who leads your tutorial will be the one marking all of your assignments, essays, and exams, and the person who gives you your final mark at the end of the year. As long as you know this piece of information, you can make it work to your advantage. Basically, you want the teaching assistant to like you and recognize that you're a hard-working individual. Here are a few tips to ensure this happens:

- **Always go to your tutorial**: Tutorials are small and teaching assistants often take attendance (especially if attendance is mandatory). Still, even if they don't take attendance, teaching assistants can easily distinguish between those students who show up regularly and those who don't. You want your teaching assistant to know that you're a hard working, serious student. Without regularly attending tutorials, the teaching assistant will never categorize you as someone worthy of an 'A'.

- **Always be prepared for tutorial**: Sometimes you'll have a reading assignment for your tutorial. Be prepared so that you can actively participate in the tutorial. Your teaching assistant will automatically recognize that you're up to date with your work.

- **Go to see your teaching assistant**: If you ever have questions, don't hesitate to see your teaching assistant. They're often more helpful than the professors who tend to explain things in a brilliant, but more complicated manner. In addition, since the teaching assistant is often the one marking all of your work, you want to make sure you do that work according to his or her guidelines. It is a good idea to bring your essays or assignments to your teaching assistant to glance over. If there is a problem, he or she will tell you about it thus enabling you to fix it before you hand it in.

- **Avoid annoying your teaching assistant**: Because tutorials are small, it can be very easy to annoy your teaching assistant. The most obvious ways to do this are by talking during class, coming in late, and being unprepared.

Remember from the beginning that teaching assistants/fellows are key in determining your final grade. You want to make a good impression. Stick to my advice and you shouldn't have any problems.

Straight A's Lesson

Teaching assistants/fellows often have significant control over your grade in a course. Take the time to form positive relationships with them and get to know what they want from you in terms of assignments, essays, and exams.

Be Prepared For Class

Unfortunately, it's not just as simple as go to class and tutorial and you'll do great in school. There are a few more things to think about than that. Obviously, one important piece of advice is that you should always be prepared for both classes and tutorials. In order to be properly prepared, you've got to bring the right things to class, do your reading ahead of time, and be awake and alert while you're there. If you do these things, you'll be in a position not only to understand what's going on in class but also to record it well in your notes.

Bring All Your Supplies To Class

You've got to have the right supplies at your fingertips to be able to concentrate and take notes appropriately. Make sure you bring the following:

- **Paper for taking notes:** In class, I use loose-leaf paper that I keep in a clipboard. At the end of the day, I remove my notes from my clipboard and store them in a three-ring binder. This method is cheap, keeps me organized, and doesn't require me to carry heavy notebooks to class.

- **Pens:** You want to bring a blue or black pen for note taking, and a red pen for underlining. Be sure that you have a few of each so you don't run out of ink during class.

- **Ruler:** Needed to underline headings in your notes.

- **Eye Glasses:** If you need glasses, never forget them when you go to class. If your eyesight is like mine, you'll be completely useless without them.

- **Handouts, Outlines, etc:** If you need any handouts, or the professor has given outlines in advance, it's a good idea to have them handy for class. They will help you follow along with the lecture.

Straight A's Lesson

To class bring paper, pens, a ruler, glasses (optional), and any handouts that are important. This way, you'll have all the supplies you need at your fingertips.

Do Your Reading Before Class

You'll probably be assigned specific readings for each class – *read them!* Here are some good reasons why you should take the time before class to do all of your required reading:

- **You'll find the lecture more interesting:** If you haven't done your reading before class, you won't have a clue what's going on. You'll be struggling throughout the lecture, trying to figure out what in the world the professor is discussing. If you already have a grasp of the material from reading it beforehand, you'll be more relaxed and more likely to find the lecture interesting and understandable.

- **You'll be able to take better notes:** If you are familiar with the terms and topics being discussed, you will be able to take better notes in class. When exam time comes, you'll be happy you have a legible and comprehensive set of notes to study from.

- **You'll be more involved in the lecture:** If you have the requisite background to the lecture, you'll be able to follow the lecture and won't feel too insecure to ask questions at opportune moments.

Overall, if you're going to take the time out of your busy schedule to attend your classes, you might as well get the most out of them by doing your reading ahead of time.

Straight A's Lesson

If you do your reading ahead of time, you'll probably find lectures to be more interesting, find it easier to take notes, and find opportune moments to ask intelligent, thought-provoking questions.

Be Awake And Alert For Class

Although you might have dragged yourself out of bed to get to class, there's really no point in catching up on your sleep once you get there. Make sure you not only go to class, but also that you pay attention. That means you've got to be up and alert. If this requires that you go to bed a little earlier at night, then do it! It's a small sacrifice that will make you so much more attentive in class.

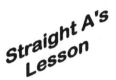 **Make sure you're alert in class so that you can concentrate. If you have to go to sleep a little earlier than you'd like to, do so.**

Being prepared for class is easy. All you've got to do is bring the right things, do your reading ahead of time and get some sleep before an early class. These are simple things that will make school success much more attainable.

Summary

This chapter has outlined some very important ideas: Go to class and tutorial, and make sure that you're prepared. If you find yourself wavering on going to class, try to think back to the reasons I've given. You've got to go to class to determine what material is the most important, to be able to predict questions on upcoming exams, and to be able to feed the professor the information he or she wants to hear on an exam. As for tutorials, remember that they are a forum where you'll get the personal attention that classes lack, you'll learn information that may show up on the exam, and you'll have an opportunity to form positive relationships with your teaching assistants/fellows (hidden gems in the marking scheme). Not only do you have to go to class and tutorials, but you also have to be properly prepared for them. You've got to bring the right things to class, make sure you've done the reading ahead of time, and be awake and alert so you can concentrate to the best of your ability. As long as you're committed to going to class and tutorials, and you're prepared for them, you'll have no problem doing well in your courses. As you'll see, the rest is easy.

CHAPTER 4

TAKE NOTES THE RIGHT WAY

Imagine yourself a week before your final exams: A little panic-stricken, perhaps? A few butterflies flitting about in your stomach? Whatever your state of mind, you'd likely feel a lot better if you had a complete, accurate, and legible set of notes to study from. Fear not, for I am giving you a simple set of instructions to keep you from pulling out the last vestiges of your hair. All you have to do is take good notes in class as well as from your textbook and the articles that you have read for class. And, there are ways to do all of this. In this chapter, I take you step-by-step through the process of taking notes in class, from textbooks, and from articles. Follow my advice and you'll have a golden set of notes to study from when exam time comes around.

Class Notes

You've conceded! You've made a pledge to yourself – and to your parents – that you'll go to class. What's next? Well, for one thing, don't assume that everything that your professor says will be magically etched into your memory through osmosis alone. You have to be prepared to take notes. And, like everything else in this book, there's a right way and a wrong way to do it.

Where To Sit

So you've made it to class – congratulations! However, before you can begin taking notes, you have to make a small but important decision: Where should you sit in that intimidating lecture hall? If your goal is to succeed in school (going back to Chapter One) then you'll want to take notes well. Being able to do this depends on finding the right seat for you in class.

Like anything else, this choice depends on a number of factors such as what type of class it is, how the professor speaks, the size of the class, whether or not you have friends in the class, etc. Finding the right seat for you in a class is often a process of trial-and-error. But, there are some general criteria that must be met for a seat to qualify as adequate.

Audibility

In the previous chapter, we established that to succeed in university, you **must** go to classes and tutorials. However, you don't have to be Einstein to realize that if you go to class and can't hear a word the professor is saying, you've defeated the purpose of being there in the first place! Going to class merely to make yourself feel like your putting in a reasonable effort just doesn't cut it. Don't waste your time. If you're not going to listen to the lectures, why even bother getting out of bed?

When you're deciding where to sit, make sure that you choose a seat where you can easily hear everything the professor is saying. Some professors refuse to use a microphone, some speak softly or too quickly, and others have a strong accent. In these classes in particular, sitting in the last row is probably not a good idea. Find a seat where you can hear what is being discussed without straining your eardrums. Somewhere in the middle of the class is usually adequate to satisfy this criterion.

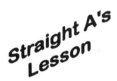

Make sure that wherever you decide to sit, you can hear everything that is being discussed during the lecture.

Visibility

While hearing the lecture is almost always the most important criteria when choosing a seat in a class, being able to see the blackboard or overheads is also extremely important. In fact, in science or math classes, being able to clearly see the blackboard might be far more important than actually hearing the lecture.

If you're in a small classroom, you probably don't have to worry about this. However, in first year, most classes tend to be rather large. Sitting at the back of the class might cause your eyes to pop out of your head as you try to copy down the formula for taking partial derivatives of a quadratic equation. Whatever the course, being able to see what is written down is not only helpful but also necessary if you want to have organized and complete notes when exam time comes.

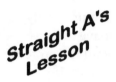 Make sure you can see what is on the blackboard or the overhead from where you sit, especially in classes that use a lot of equations and formulas.

Comfort

You're probably thinking: "It's pretty obvious that you should sit in a seat where you'll be able to see and hear what is going on in the lecture." Nevertheless, it is tempting to find a seat at the back of the class with a large group of your friends and socialize. School can definitely be more enjoyable when you listen to a lecture with a group of your friends. And, there is something to be said for sitting with friends in a class. It's comforting. Being in college can be an intimidating experience at times and having a group of friends nearby always makes you feel a little more at ease. It might not be a bad idea to consider having a comforting place to sit in a class.

Still, you've got to remember your ultimate goal – achievement! If you want to achieve your goals, you should think about:

1. Who you are choosing to sit with, and
2. What your learning style is.

If you're the kind of person who needs to have absolutely no distractions in order to follow the lecture, then it's probably a better idea for you to find a seat in an area away from anyone who may distract you. On the other hand, you might be the kind of person that finds it helpful to sit with friends. That way, when you miss a word or a line you can just lean over their shoulder and get some help. Wherever you choose to sit, keep in mind that you dragged yourself out of bed to get to class. Don't waste your time by not paying attention. Sit somewhere where you can both listen and see. And if the people around you are going to distract you, find a better spot.

The exact seat you choose really isn't that important as long as you've satisfied the three criteria: You must be able to hear the lecture, see what's going on, and feel comfortable where you are.

Once you've found that right seat, even if it's taken a few classes to pinpoint it, try to hold onto it. Well, obviously you're not literally going to be able to hold onto the seat from class to class, never allowing anyone else to sit in it. But trying to sit in the same general area, class after class is a good idea for two reasons. First, since people generally tend to sit in the same area in a class, it's likely you'll become friends with the people that sit around you; and second, keeping your seat from class to class creates a consistent routine for you. This will allow you to concentrate more on taking notes and listening to your lecture. You may even find that it helps you to learn from and remember the lecture better when you sit in the same area and at the same distance from the professor and blackboard.

A reliable system is needed to do well in college. Sitting in the right seat, and continuing to do so class after class will keep you on the right track.

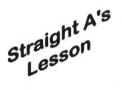 Find a seat where you feel relaxed but alert. Get into the habit of going back to that seat class after class.

What To Listen For

In some of your classes it may seem as though you're eavesdropping on a private conversation between your professor and himself about something you haven't a clue about. The reality is that while your professor may be brilliant in his particular specialty, he may not be so adept at presentation. This is the worst-case scenario. Hopefully though, you'll find that the majority of your professors will have something important to talk about and will do so in a logical and organized manner. Having a coherent professor will make taking notes a fairly straightforward task. Regardless of who your lecturer is or what his or her lecturing abilities may be however, it's still possible for you to take good notes by learning the skills of this art. It's helpful to think of note taking as your responsibility and not your professors'. Get a handle on what to do to ensure that your notes will be up to par.

Write Down All The Essentials

You might initially laugh at the person next to you who frantically scribbles his or her notes during class and doesn't talk to anybody. However, you certainly won't even snicker when it comes to exam time and you're begging that person to lend you their class notes. Who's laughing now?

While I myself avoid frantically writing down every word the professor says in class, I do tend to take a lot of notes. Sure, just listening to a lecture without taking notes can give you a good grasp of the content. But the fact is that if you have five classes a week with each class meeting two or three times, you're attending way too many lectures to remember which professor said what in which class and on which day. When it comes down to exam time, what do you have to go by? Can you really trust your memory to store and recall all that information?

On a personal note, I can't rely on my memory alone. As a result, I take a lot of notes. That way, I have a complete and accurate set of notes when the time comes to study. Also, the physical act of writing ideas down on paper helps some people to actually remember things better.

Writing down what is being taught can also keep your mind focused on what is going on in class for those of you whose minds have a tendency to wander. This can keep you actively engaged in class and ready to offer intelligent questions and comments on the material.

Be active! Pick up a pen and get to work. It will help you learn the material now and will give you comprehensive notes to study from when you need them.

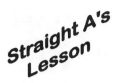

Be active in class. Write a lot of notes so that you learn the material now and have a complete set of notes to study from during exam time.

This does not mean that you have to be hanging on every word the professor says. However, you should definitely include in your notes all of the main points plus any examples and useful material that the professor discusses. This task seems so complicated now but when you know exactly what to listen for, deciphering the real important stuff from the moderately important stuff will be easy.

Use Short Hand

It's not possible to write every word out in full if you want to keep up with the pace of most lectures. To be adept at taking notes in class, it's important that you are a quick note taker. This usually requires the use of some form of shorthand.

Don't worry … I'm not going to recommend you enroll in some classes to learn how to take proper shorthand. Only *you* need to understand your notes, so you can come up with your very own system of shorthand.

I'll give you some tips to create your own shorthand. However, you can trust that your own unique shorthand will evolve naturally while you're taking notes in your classes.

- **Vowels:** A quick way to shorten words in your notes is to cut out a bunch of vowels. Words are still pretty recognizable this way. For example, *could* becomes *cld*, *around* changes to *arnd*, and *computers* is *cmpters*. Be careful not to make words unrecognizable though. For example, you shouldn't write *plce* for *police*, because you could mistake it for another word like *place*. You'll get the hang of it as you go along.

- **Common Words:** Most people have simple short forms for common words. In addition to the symbols I show you below, I strongly suggest that you make up your own symbols for words that are repeated often in your notes (you can get started by trying out the exercise at the end of this section):

Because – b/c	Therefore - $\therefore$
At - @	Number - #
More than - >	Less than - <
Increasing - ↑	Decreasing - ↓
Which – wh	Approximately/About - $\cong$
Same as - =	Following – ff
Resulting in - →	As a consequence of / As a result of- ←
Change - Δ	Compare; In Comparison – cf
And - +	

- **Endings:** Shortening the ends of words is a great time saver. For example, in words that end with *ion*, just write an *n*. That way, words such as *repetition*, *competition*, and *superstition*, are reduced to *repetitn*, *competitn*, and *superstitn*.

- **Beginnings:** Get into the habit of just writing down the beginning of some words. For example, you can write *esp* instead of *especially*.

- **????:** There will be points in your lectures where you are confused and want to ask someone for an explanation at a later time. Simply jot down a bunch of question marks around this problematic material to indicate that you don't completely understand what you wrote down.

- ******:** When the professor says something that you know is important (either because he says it is or because you just have a feeling that it is), indicate its significance with a bunch of asterisks.

- **Indicate 'Possible Exam Question' (PEQ):** During a lecture, your professor might say something like, "Don't be surprised if you get a question about this on your exam!" This information is very important to jot down. Write down PEQ next to the material whenever your professor says something of that nature.

Straight A's Lesson   **Make up your own shorthand so that you're able to take in-depth notes at a fast pace.**

Listen For Headings

To keep your notes organized, you've got to write down *headings*. What are headings? They are the topics that will be discussed, similar to chapters in a book. They indicate the focus of the lecture and help you decipher what the professor will be talking about and when he will be talking about it. There are three different types of headings: **Main headings, sub-headings,** and **categorical headings.** All are equally important and you've got to pay attention to them to follow the lecture and take notes properly.

Main Heading: At the beginning of each lecture, most professors will write on the board (or perhaps say out loud) what the topic is they will be discussing. This is often the title of the lecture. We'll refer to this as the *main heading*. It should be written at the top of a fresh piece of paper and underlined. This is the overall focus of the lecture and it should be made clear in your notes.

If you're lucky, you may have a professor who is highly organized and he or she might bring overheads to class that list the topics that will be discussed during the day's lecture. If not, you'll have to organize your notes for yourself. This is a little more complicated but certainly not worthy of panic.

Sub-headings: Once you have a *main heading* for the lecture, you're on your way. The next things to concern yourself with are *sub-headings*. For example, the professor may be discussing Shakespeare's poetry in a certain lecture. This would be the main heading of the lecture. Once the professor begins to lecture, you realize that he or she is planning to discuss the various types of poetry Shakespeare wrote such as sonnets, ballads, etc. In this case, 'Shakespeare's Poetry' would be the main heading for the lecture and the different types of poetry (such as 'Shakespeare's Sonnets') would each be a *sub-heading*. As you can see, the main heading is the most general description of the lecture topic. The next level of headings – the sub-headings – are more specific. Next, we'll look at categorical headings, which are even more topic-specific than sub-headings.

Categorical Headings: Continuing with the Shakespeare example, suppose that in discussing the different types of poetry, the professor presents examples of specific Shakespearean works. The title of each poetic example can be thought of as *categorical headings* and should be clearly marked in your notes. Categorical headings are even more specific than sub-headings and get to the core of what the professor is discussing.

You should now have some idea about the differences between main headings, sub-headings, and categorical headings. The easiest way to understand the three types of headings and their relation to one another is by arranging them in an upside-down pyramid. As you move towards the bottom of the pyramid, headings become more narrow and specific.

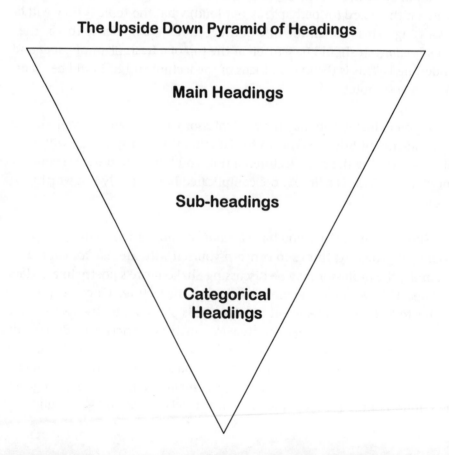

The Upside Down Pyramid of Headings

Main Headings

Sub-headings

Categorical Headings

Differentiate Your Headings: It's important in your notes that you differentiate the various types of headings from one another. You want to be able to easily distinguish between your main heading, sub-headings, and categorical headings. The easiest way to do this is by creating a pattern that indicates the different types of headings. Here's the pattern that I use (but feel free to choose your own pattern if you like):

- Use two red lines to underline the main heading at the top of your page.
- Use one red line for subheadings.
- Use two black or blue lines for categorical headings.
- For other headings that are even more specific, use one black or blue line.

Whatever method you choose to use, the important thing to keep in mind is that each level of headings should be marked in the same way. That way, your notes are easy to read and are clearly divided into sections that you can conquer one at a time when you buckle down to study for exams. All of this organization will not be in vain. When exam time comes, you'll be prepared with a complete and organized set of notes to work from.

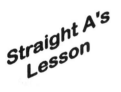

Straight A's Lesson

Don't underestimate the importance of structure in your notes. Create your own system for indicating main headings, sub-headings, and categorical headings and stick to this system in all of your classes.

Listen For Summary Points

Everything the professor says is fair game and potential exam material. However, not everything he or she says is equally important. You've got to keep this in mind when listening to a lecture.

In most lectures, professors will have a fundamental message they want to convey. They are giving you a broad range of information and material to make a point about something they consider important. Hopefully the point of the lecture will be obvious. If so, get it down into your notes – pronto!

Here's an example to illustrate what I mean. You're in a sociology class discussing various social problems. For the entire lecture, the professor gives you examples and information about the media. She shows you how the media portrayed a civil war in Africa and how it covered riots in Washington. It becomes apparent that the media maintains a powerful control over the way we, the public, view social problems. Okay ... you've got the *point!*

Your professor will almost always have a central point to a lecture. This will be expressed throughout the lecture several times, possibly presented in a different way each time. Occasionally, the professor may not articulate it at all. No matter what though, you should be listening for it and writing down in your notes your version of the basic idea of the lecture. This point, I'll refer to as a **summary point**. It's what the professor is really trying to get across. In other words, it's kind of like the thesis of a lecture; that is, what is being proven by the professor.

In high school, you learn a lot of facts. In university, your education is raised to a new level. Here you are encouraged to compile related facts into a reasonable argument. This is exactly what your professors are doing during each lecture. They have a summary point they want to convey to their students. They do so by giving facts and information that lead up to the summary point.

You've got to know summary points for three important reasons:

- **Organization**: To be able to organize your notes properly, you need to know the point of the lecture, or the summary point. That way, you can differentiate the summary point from the information/facts presented by the professor.

- **Understanding**: In order to understand the lecture, it helps to know the significance of what the professor is saying. The significance of the lecture relates to the summary point, or what the professor is trying to convey. If you miss this summary point, it's likely you missed the heart of the lecture.

- **Exam Preparation**: A common question on written exams is as follows: Explain 'x' and state the significance of it.

Explaining 'x' will require that you know the facts/information that were presented in class. The significance of 'x' usually lies in the summary point: What were all of these facts leading to? When you study, you want to make sure that you have a good handle on the summary points.

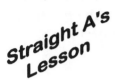

Listen for summary points, that is, what the professor is trying to prove in his or her lecture. This helps you to effectively organize the material in your notes.

Exercise

Develop Your Own Shorthand

In the left-hand column below, write down two dozen words that you find are frequently repeated in your notes. Then, either by using the suggestions I have given, or by coming up with your own, write down a shorter form of the word in the right hand column. This will help you to develop your own system of shorthand. You can also use this list as a reference sheet if you find you're having trouble keeping up with the pace of class lectures.

Full Word	Shorter Form		Full Word	Shorter Form
1. _____	_____		13. _____	_____
2. _____	_____		14. _____	_____
3. _____	_____		15. _____	_____
4. _____	_____		16. _____	_____
5. _____	_____		17. _____	_____
6. _____	_____		18. _____	_____
7. _____	_____		19. _____	_____
8. _____	_____		20. _____	_____
9. _____	_____		21. _____	_____
10. _____	_____		22. _____	_____
11. _____	_____		23. _____	_____
12. _____	_____		24. _____	_____

Textbook Notes

In most of your classes, you'll have a fairly large textbook from which you are required to read specific sections. So, in addition to taking class notes, you've also got to know what to do with this textbook material. Do you take notes? If so, how detailed do you get and how much time should you dedicate to this kind of material? All of these questions will be answered.

Be Up To Date In Your Reading

The textbook is usually a supplement to the class material. It is supposed to help you understand what you're doing in class and give you more detailed information on the topics discussed in lecture. I'll give you a method that you should follow to keep up with textbook material and then, I'll give you a second method in case you find yourself pressed for time.

Textbook Method #1: Read the textbook material before the class in which it will be discussed. Then, after the lecture, take notes on the textbook. This method:

- Familiarizes you with the material before you go to class, making it easier for you to take notes on the topic during the lecture;

- Gives you a perspective on the material for when you attend lecture, making it easier to distinguish what information in lecture is central and what information is of secondary importance;

- Makes taking notes on the textbook after the lecture simple because you can sift through the textbook and determine what material you should be concentrating on (i.e. that material that the professor highlights in class).

Textbook Method #2: If you really can't find the time to read the textbook before you go to class and take notes afterwards, it is possible to merge the two steps into one. How do you do this? Before you go to class, take notes on the textbook material. Taking notes on textbook material before you attend lecture is a little more complicated because you won't have a handle on what information is the most important and what information you shouldn't even bother writing down. In fact, you may end up taking notes on a lot of useless material. You may also skip over some information that you realize is fairly important after you've attended the lecture. To ensure your notes are accurate, you might have to add some information after the lecture by going back to your textbook. Nevertheless, using this method will still prepare you for class with the textbook material already read.

Regardless of which textbook method you use, the most important thing to remember is that you really must be up to date with your readings. Don't decide that reading the textbook is a waste of time or just doesn't fit into your schedule! Eventually, you'll have to sit down with this large textbook and read it. Come the week before your exam, you just won't have enough time to do it.

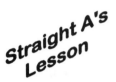 Be consistent and take notes from your textbook on a day-to-day basis so that you're up to date with your class. By the time the exam rolls around, you'll have a complete set of textbook notes from which to study.

Know What To Read Vs. What To Take Notes On

Reading a textbook is very different from taking notes from one. If you have enough time, it's best to separate each stage and follow Textbook Method #1 as outlined above (i.e. read the textbook material first and then go back and take your notes after you've attended the lecture).

Whichever textbook method you choose however, you should know that the techniques for reading a textbook differ from the techniques you should use when taking notes from one.

Reading A Textbook:

- Understand the textbook: Follow along with each line that you read and try to understand the information as it is given.

- Get interested in the information: Try to actually enjoy what you're reading and get immersed in it. Instead of reading for pure content, try to see the bigger picture of what is being said and discussed.

Straight A's Lesson

Read the textbook slow enough so that you understand all the material in it. Try to immerse yourself deeply in the material in order to find the information interesting and worthwhile.

Taking Notes From The Textbook:

- Get to the point: Reading is for interest; note taking is for exam preparation. When you take notes you want to get the point – and fast! You want to write down only that information that will be pertinent to the exam.

- Be thorough: While you want to get to the point when you're taking notes from a textbook, you also want to be thorough enough so that you won't have to refer back to your textbook when it's time to study for your exam.

- See the textbook as a supplement to the class lectures: When taking notes from a textbook, you want to concentrate on the information that sheds light on lecture discussions. Thinking of the textbook as a supplement to class material makes it easier to determine what you should be writing down in your notes.

- Different classes require different textbook methods: Usually, the textbook is a supplement to the class material. Sometimes, however, the professor will assign you a chapter that he or she is not planning to discuss during lecture. Clearly, when you take notes on this chapter, you'll want to be more comprehensive than when you take notes on a chapter that you've discussed during a lecture. Keep in mind that each class requires a different technique of note taking and adjust your routine accordingly.

Straight A's Lesson

When taking notes from textbooks, try to leave out useless material while making sure that you've written down any pertinent information. Be picky when you take notes and think about what is really going to be important when you study for your upcoming exam.

Don't Get Bogged Down

As has already been noted, a lot of the time a textbook is merely a *supplement* to the class lectures. Because the textbook provides a tremendous amount of information, much of which is beyond the scope of the class, it usually is not required that you understand and memorize it word for word. So don't get bogged down by a lot of extraneous information in the textbook. The point of reading and taking notes from a textbook is to be consistent on a day-to-day basis. This will help you become familiar with the class material. If you get bogged down with unimportant parts of the reading, you're not going to have enough time to finish the rest of your reading. While you're getting stuck with minute details, you'll likely be missing the important material in the textbook that has a chance of showing up on an exam.

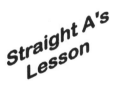

Straight A's Lesson

Don't get bogged down by textbook material. Do your best by keeping up to date by taking notes on your readings.

Taking Notes From Articles

In many of your classes, you'll probably get a reader full of articles that you'll be required to read. Many of these articles will deal with topics similar to the ones you've dealt with in class. However, most articles present topics from a specific point of view (i.e. the author's).

Article material is generally very different from textbook reading. Whereas textbook material is largely bias-free, most articles are written to prove a thesis. Because textbooks and articles are inherently different, reading them and taking notes from them will also require a fairly different process. There is a system for reading an article and taking notes from it that will ensure that you've extracted all of its important details. Read on!

The Full Read

When you read a textbook you are usually extracting a lot of facts and information from it. Reading an article, on the other hand, is not about reading facts. While facts are presented in an article, these facts are included for a very specific reason: To support the author's argument or explain a point the article is making.

With a textbook, it is possible (but not the best strategy) to take notes during your first read (see Textbook Method #2). On the other hand, when you read an article, taking notes without first fully reading the article in depth is a useless endeavor. You've got to get a handle on the information before worrying about how you are going to take notes on it.

The first step when you are assigned articles to read for class is to read the articles the whole way through, underlining any important points as you go. (I'll give you some advice on what you should be underlining in the next section.)

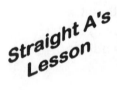

When you get an article for class, before you can take notes on it you have to sit down and read the whole article from beginning to end.

Divide The Article

To be able to understand an article, you should recognize the typical format:

- **Introduction:** Typically, articles begin with an introduction. In the introduction, the author gives some general comments relating to the topic and then presents the thesis statement or statement of intent. That is, what the article is trying to prove or explain.

- **Body:** The body of the article is dedicated to proving the thesis. This may include statistics, personal anecdotes, or theoretical information. It also may include showing other points of view and picking apart any support for these views.

- **Conclusion:** The article usually ends with a restatement of the thesis and some remarks that speak of the argument's significance in a larger context.

Understanding this structure makes analyzing an article much easier. When you read an article for the first time, highlight or underline certain points according to the following guidelines:

- In the introduction, underline the thesis and make sure you understand it. (Be sure to look up any words that you're not too sure about.)

- In the body of the article, underline the main points that prove the thesis. Try to pick out the main points the author is making rather than underlining the explanations or elements of proof.

- In the conclusion of the article, underline the restatement of the thesis (if there is one) and the comments that the author makes that reflect the significance of the argument in a larger context.

Now that you've underlined the article's main points and you've read it carefully to understand it, it's time to take notes on the article. Taking notes on the article will be simple because you've already done the hard part ... you've worked on understanding the article in the first place. You just have to record what you've learned so you have it handy when studying for your exams.

Here's what you do when taking notes on articles:

- Write down the thesis. Quote the author by using his or her words and then write it down in your own words to make sure you've got it.

- Write down the main points the author makes to prove the thesis.

- Under each main point the author makes, write down at least three points (the more you write down the better) that the author uses to support these main points.

- Focus on what the author is trying to prove rather than specific details. If you have to read a bunch of articles, there is no way you'll be tested on specific details in each one. But, you should know the basic facts presented and what these facts are leading the author to conclude.

Straight A's Lesson   **When you take notes on an article, be sure to write down the thesis of the article and the proof the author presents to support his or her thesis.**

Evaluate The Article

When you read an article, you're really trying to develop a perspective on an argument, controversy, or theory. If you've read it thoroughly and taken notes appropriately, you should be able to think about one last thing – your own evaluation of the article. Do you think that the author proved what he or she set out to prove?

You will most likely discuss this article at some point in class or at a conference with a teaching assistant or teaching fellow. If you've read the article thoroughly, taken notes from it according to the guidelines I set out, and spent time thinking about it in order to give your own personal evaluation, you'll be in a good position to discuss the article in detail.

Straight A's Lesson   **When you are assigned articles to read in a class, first fully read the article before you attempt to take notes on it. When taking notes, make sure you've written down the thesis of the article, the main points the author is making, and any facts that help explain the main points. After you've finished taking notes, try to do your own evaluation of the article in terms of how well the argument was supported and how believable the article was.**

Keeping Yourself Organized During The School Year

You'll have a lot of things going on during the year: Assignments and essays due, exams to write, classes to attend, tutorials to prepare for, and many other activities I don't have space here to list. Your head just can't handle trying to remember all the different dates, times, and places you'll need to know.

That's why it's crucial that you keep yourself organized during the year by keeping an agenda or planner. You'll want to have a handy organizer in which you write down everything you have to do during the day, and any days on which you have something to hand in or have some place that you're supposed to be.

Here are some tricks to remember on keeping an organized agenda:

- **Put in red boxes anything that is crucial to remember**: For example, make a box around entries like 'Hand in English essay' and 'Economics mid-term at 2:00 p.m.'. These are the kind of things that you absolutely do not want to risk forgetting.

- **When you complete something in your agenda, highlight it**: It will satisfy you at the end of the day to go through your agenda highlighting all the things you've accomplished. Highlighting is much better than crossing out because you'll still be able to see what you've written down and you might need the information at a later date.

- **Keep up to date with your agenda**: You should write things into your agenda every day as they come up. For example, as soon as you're assigned a paper to hand in, mark the due date in your agenda. You'll also have to go through your agenda every night to see what you have and haven't accomplished for the day.

- **Make deadlines for yourself in your agenda**: If you decide you want to finish all the reading for a certain course a week from now, you should write it down in your agenda. You'll take the deadline more seriously if you keep coming across it in your agenda.

- **Preview your week on Sundays**: Every Sunday night before you begin your school week, look over your agenda to see what you have upcoming. This will help you to get your mind set on accomplishing all of your tasks for the week.

- **Keep your agenda handy**: It's a good idea to have an agenda that isn't too big or bulky and that you don't mind carrying with you most of the time. Having it with you in class or in the library will allow you to write down things as you think of them.

- **Trick yourself**: Sometimes, I'll write in my agenda that an assignment is due a few days before it actually is so I'll be sure to have it done well in advance. If you're the kind of person that waits until the last minute to complete assignments and essays, trick yourself by writing in false dates (but still record somewhere when the actual essay is due). This will allow you more time than you are used to having. Now you'll be able to do the last minute corrections or touch ups to your essays or assignments that you never had the time for previously.

Completing Assignments And Exercises

Throughout the year, in addition to essays (discussed in Chapter Nine) you'll probably have assignments and exercises to hand in. This occurs most frequently in math, science, economics, engineering, and other such classes. Here's what to do when you get these assignments:

- **Don't delay:** Some assignments will be tedious and time consuming. When they are assigned, it's best to start them right away to ensure you'll have enough time to complete them properly.

- **Finish the required reading beforehand**: Assignments usually test whether you've done the required reading or have been listening to class lectures. Don't try to do the assignments without actually learning the material first!

- **Do them by yourself, then compare with others**: Assignments are given to help you understand what you're learning in class. To really understand the material, you want to try to figure out assignments for yourself. Only once you've finished the assignment on your own should you compare your answers with others to see if they're correct.

- **Make sure your answers are correct**: You want to make sure that you're handing in a close-to-perfect assignment. There really is no reason why you should be losing marks on assignments that you had a long time to complete. I suggest going to whatever lengths to make sure you're answering the questions correctly. You might want to get help on assignments by talking to your teaching assistant/fellow or your professor. If the assignment is particularly difficult, you might even think of hiring a tutor (possibly sharing the cost with other classmates) to go over your answers before you hand the assignment in.

- **Correct your assignments**: Once your assignment is handed back, don't put it on the shelf and assume that you'll never have to look at it again. The material on the assignments will more than likely show up on a future exam. For that reason, you want to make sure that you correct any questions that you got wrong by either getting help from a classmate or by going to see the professor. That way, when exam time comes, you'll have accurate assignments from which to study.

Commonly Asked Questions

Question: Should I tape the lectures and then listen to them later to take notes?

Answer: I strongly suggest that you don't. Taping lectures is a waste of time. You already have too many classes and too much else to do at university. You just don't have the time to listen to each lecture twice. With the tactics that were presented earlier in this chapter, you should be able to take complete and accurate notes during the actual lecture. If for some reason you really can't take lecture notes quickly enough (perhaps because of a medical condition, or language barrier), only then should you resort to taping your lectures and listening to them later.

Question: If the course notes are sold at the bookstore, do I still need to take notes during lectures?

Answer: Yes. Just because you can buy notes that were written by someone else doesn't mean that you're off the hook and don't need to take class notes yourself. As I've said before, class notes tend to be the most important study aids once exam time comes. You want to make sure that you have as accurate notes as possible. You can only ensure this if you sit there and take notes yourself – notes that you trust! In addition, taking notes in class helps you follow along with the lecture and learn the material much more thoroughly. Don't dismiss note taking right away.

It's great if you have the opportunity to buy the notes for a class. A lot of times these are transcribed word for word. However, combining these notes with those that you took on your own is really the best thing you can do.

Question: How many hours should I be working each night while I'm in school?

Answer: Some books will tell you that you should be studying a specific amount of time each night. For example, I've read that you should work between 1 ½ to 2 hours for each hour of class that you attend. Personally, I am against giving this kind of advice. Instead, I think you should be as efficient as possible in school. That means, you should get the most amount of work done in the shortest period of time. It's not how long you study, it's the quality of the studying done.

My suggestion is that you set goals for yourself about what you plan to get accomplished during each week. You want to have all of your class reading done ahead of time and then take notes on the your readings after the lectures. However long this takes you is as long as you should be working during the week. There's no doubt that it is a bit time-consuming, but remember that you are at school to succeed. Stick it out and try to fulfill your academic goals.

Summary

Congratulations! You now have a strong understanding of how to take notes the proper way. You can go to class with no problem, read and take notes from a textbook, and also understand articles like a true academic. If you are consistent in taking complete and accurate notes during the year, you should end up at exam time with an unbelievably organized set of notes to study from. However, taking notes is the easy part. The difficult part is making sure that you do it consistently on a day-to-day basis throughout the year both in class and from your readings at home.

CHAPTER 5

NETWORK

Imagine that you've just found out you've won a huge lottery and there's no one around for you to tell. Or, imagine that you're lost in a strange city and there's nobody in sight to ask for directions. There are a lot of situations where having the right people around can be very helpful. Being in university is definitely one of them.

At university, there are people everywhere you turn. This is a good thing. Getting to know these people and being able to get advice and help from them when you need it is what this chapter is all about. Simply put: You've got to learn how to network.

There are three groups of people you want to make sure that you form solid and positive relationships with. The first group is your classmates; becoming friends with your classmates can make attending class so much more enjoyable and can really help you succeed in your courses. I refer to the second group as 'older students'; students who are a few years ahead of you hold valuable information and advice that you can really benefit from. Finally, there are your professors and your teaching assistants/fellows; developing and maintaining positive relationships with them can come in handy throughout the semester. For example, if your mark in a class borders between two grades, this final group holds the power to bump it up depending on how they feel about you as a student. Learning how to create positive relationships throughout your university years with these three groups of people is the goal of this chapter.

Classmates

You attend so many classes and there are so many people in each one. Do you have to be best friends with everyone in your class? Is that even a good idea? What kind of relationships should you develop with your classmates anyway? While there really are no right answers, let me give you some suggestions that have worked for me from year to year.

Find A Study Buddy

Clearly, knowing people in your classes is important. That doesn't mean that you have to know the names and phone numbers of every one of your classmates. However, you should have at least one person with whom you feel comfortable enough to call and even work with from time to time. That person can be a lifesaver when you have to return home for a family event or when you come down with a fever and can't make it to class for a few days. More assuring is the knowledge that you can call that person with questions about an assignment or upcoming exam. It's imperative that you know a person in each of your classes that you can contact with any questions or from whom you can borrow notes when you miss a class.

My grade two teacher used to refer to this type of person as a "study buddy". However, it can't just be any Tom, Dick, or Harry. Your "study buddy" should have the following specific characteristics:

- **Attends class regularly**: If your "study buddy" doesn't attend class regularly, then there is obviously no point in calling him or her to find out what you've missed in class. Chances are that they didn't attend either.

- **Takes good class notes**: The notes that your "study buddy" takes must be comprehensive enough so that you can understand them, and legible enough so that you can read them.

- **A conscientious student**: Your "study buddy" should be up-to-date with his or her work. That way, when you have questions you want to ask about the class material, he or she will be able to help you out.

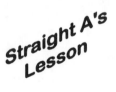

Make sure you have at least one person in every class that you can rely on to ask questions of and get notes from when you miss a class.

Be Friendly – But Not Too Friendly

People in your class can be an excellent source of help. For example, some of your classmates will have older brothers and sisters who have taken the same classes and have a complete set of notes, old exams and midterms. Other classmates will be blessed with a remarkable understanding of the subject matter and can be helpful when you have assignments that you just don't understand. For purely practical reasons then, it's good to be friendly with many people in your class. As well, forming positive relationships with them can make your classes more enjoyable and comfortable. Remember: Friendliness pays off in a class atmosphere!

A word of caution here: Being 'too friendly' with your classmates or with friends outside of your classes, can sometimes work against you. If you're at school to achieve your best, you've got to know how to set boundaries with others and be able to say 'no'. This is easier than it may sound. Let me give you some likely scenarios you might encounter and some ways in which to deal with them:

- **Example #1**: A friend in your class wants to photocopy all of your notes the night before the exam. You couldn't be more annoyed because you've got your own studying to do and don't want to worry about getting your notes back in time. Don't hesitate to give a firm 'no' to this request. The night before the exam (or better yet, the last few nights before the exam), all you should be concerning yourself with is how *you* are going to do. Anyone who has waited until the last minute and has no notes to study from is irresponsible and you should not feel committed to help them.

- **Example #2**: Your friend has not stopped calling you, asking every question imaginable about your upcoming calculus final. You didn't mind it the first few times; in fact, you were a bit flattered. But, know when enough is enough! You've got your own studying to do. Simply tell your friend you're busy studying and if that person is a true friend, he or she will appreciate your need for a little space before the exam. Besides, you're setting the example for them to do likewise when other people ask too much of them.

There are many more examples I could cite. These are just two to emphasize how many favors will be asked of you by others in school (especially now that you are a successful student). Personally, I have tried my best to help those who've asked for assistance and I have found many of my good gestures reciprocated in turn. But it took me a little while to discover just where I had to draw the line. You must determine just how much help you're comfortable giving to others. Keep in mind that the only mark you really have to worry about is your own. You must be able to say no – and do so with confidence – when you feel it's warranted. Besides, no one respects a pushover.

Saying no to classmates is one thing; saying no to friends is much more difficult. For instance, you might really want to go to that frat party the night before your American Lit midterm and your friends might be pressuring you to go. However, as we're beginning to understand, doing well in school requires setting priorities and sticking to them. In this case, you'll just have to say no so that you'll be at your best for your midterm.

Straight A's Lesson

Being friendly with classmates in university is a good idea, but you've also got to be able to draw the line when requests are too difficult to carry out. Put your own needs and goals before those of your friends or classmates when it comes down to it.

Don't Waste Your Time With Study Groups

In my opinion, study groups can give you the sense that you're accomplishing something when, in reality, you're just going for coffee with a bunch of friends. Study groups are extremely popular in undergrad around exam time. Groups of students will meet at the coffee shop in the student area or at someone's apartment the night before exams and will rationalize that they're getting a lot of work done. Don't waste your time. Study groups are almost always unproductive. Here are three reasons why you shouldn't waste your time in study groups:

1. You have to rely on yourself to learn the information – You have a great deal of information to learn for a class. While discussing it with friends may familiarize you with this information, when you actually go into the exam, your friends won't be there to write it for you. You're going to be the one with a pen in your hand and a blank page in front of you. Often in study groups, you're just listening to other people reciting what they know. And while some of this information may be absorbed, it's much more efficient to use your time to study the material on your own using the study method that I will present in Chapter Seven.

2. Study groups lack structure – In a study group, there is often no system in place as to how to go over the material in a logical and coherent manner. With several people convening, it's very hard to find an efficient way to put all of the material together. Instead, what ends up happening is that the material is examined in a haphazard way. Important information is not dealt with properly while insignificant information tends to be over-analyzed.

3. Study groups are merely forums for people who want to show off – Once they've learned the course material, many students like to boost their confidence by showing off what they know in a group environment. They can easily answer all of the questions thrown their way and they feel confident they've done a decent job of studying. Short of being a forum for the display of one's knowledge, however, study groups are a waste of time (and, listening to someone else boast of their knowledge might derail your own confidence).

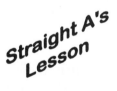

Study the course material primarily on your own. Study groups are often a waste of valuable time.

Older Students

When I use the term 'older students' (not to be confused with 'mature students'), I am referring to students who are a few years ahead of you in school. These students tend to be an underutilized resource at university. It's a little known fact that these students can be very useful for several things including providing you with notes, dispensing advice on your classes, and giving you the scoop about various professors. They've already 'been there and done that' and as a result, they may have some insight that you lack. Unfortunately, many students just don't realize the advantages of getting to know them.

Get To Know Older Students

Getting to know older students is not as difficult as it might first appear. Even if you don't know anyone who fits this description, there are many ways you can connect with older students. Here are a few suggestions:

- **Classmate Connections:** If you're friendly with people in your class, then you probably know someone with an older brother or sister, or someone who has a friend a few years ahead of you.

- **Older Students In Your Class:** You'll probably have a few people in each of your classes who are a year or two ahead of you and are just taking that class because they were studying abroad or couldn't fit it into their schedules in previous years. These people will probably have taken other classes that you too may soon be taking. Simply being in the same class as them is an easy way to get to know them. You might be able to help them in the class that you take with them, and in return, they might be able to help you in classes you're about to take.

- **Clubs:** Joining clubs in your faculty or getting involved in student body politics will introduce you to all sorts of students, many of whom can be helpful in giving you useful advice.

- **Faculty Social Events:** At my school, and I'm sure many others, there are occasionally faculty gatherings such as a "wine and cheese" or "beer and pizza" events. Although you might not feel like going to these, they might be useful because they can give you an opportunity to meet the people in your faculty who are a few years ahead of you.

If you make an effort, you should have no problem meeting older students. Knowing these people is a good idea so that you can ask them for help and advice.

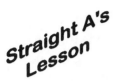 **Meeting older students is easy to do. Get to know them through your classmates, by getting involved in clubs or school politics, or by attending faculty events.**

Ask Older Students For Help And Advice

Once you've met some older students, you can take the opportunity to ask them for help. Initially, you may feel intimidated by them or feel that you'll be viewed as an annoyance. Don't sweat it! People love to display their expertise. When you ask them for advice, they'll be flattered and more than happy to help you out.

You'll need to know what kind of information you're looking for from older students. Even more important than getting valuable information about classes and professors from them, is getting your hands on past midterms and final exams that they may have. (Just make sure this is legal!) Before you approach a midterm or final exam, you want to have a solid idea of what kind of questions you can expect. One of the best ways to know this is to review past exams that have been given by your professor.

In the next chapter, I discuss how to use these past exams. For now, however, remember that throughout the term – and even before the term begins – you should get your resources in order. Make sure that you've tapped all of your resources to try to get your hands on past exams and midterms.

There are often past exams on reserve at the university library. If your older student friends can't help you out, go to the library and inquire about past exams even if the professor hasn't mentioned that they're available.

Meet older students. They can give you advice on classes and professors and, more importantly, give you past exams to study from.

Don't Let Older Students Scare You

If you do end up meeting some older students, there is one thing to be wary of: Some of them may purposely try to scare you by telling you how awful a certain professor is or perhaps how difficult a certain class that you are required to take is. They might say something like, "Don't even bother trying to do well in that class – it's impossible!" My advice here is not to pay any attention to these comments. As I've stressed throughout this book, as long as you have a system of doing well in university, you can obtain a top mark in any class.

When students tried to throw me off course with such remarks, instead of getting frightened or intimidated, I took a different approach. Quite simply, I set out to prove them wrong. I decided to demonstrate to these unfortunate students that while they might have found it impossible to do well, I was going to find my own way to succeed. Sure, you're supposed to do well for your own sake, but once in a while it's fun to prove someone wrong. And hey, if it ends up forcing you to do better in a course, then why not?

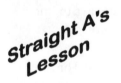

Don't ever let older students intimidate you with tales of impossible classes and scary professors. Instead, prove them wrong by showing them that what they thought was an impossible class wasn't so impossible after all.

Professors And Teaching Assistants/Fellows

These are the people who teach you, answer your questions, and post your final grade in a course. Building good relations with these power figures is something you want to take seriously. Why? Well, besides the fact that they'll be able to write good reference letters for you, they can also bump you up or down a percentage point or two if you are bordering on a grade in a course. If they like you, they'll probably raise your grade.

The Division Of Power Between Professors And Teaching Assistants/Fellows

We all know that being liked by your professors is a really good thing. Fewer people, however, recognize the real hidden gem in the marking scheme: The teaching assistants or teaching fellows (see Chapter Three). In many of the classes you take, the teaching assistant will be the one submitting your mark. The professor will likely not even discuss it with them. Therefore, getting to know your teaching assistant/fellow is just as important, if not more so, than getting to know your professor.   I want to stress that you should never overlook the importance of teaching assistants in controlling your grade in any given course.

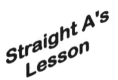

Teaching assistants often have more control over your course grade than the professor does. Don't overlook their importance and try to establish good relationships with them.

Form Good Relations With Professors And Teaching Assistants/Fellows

Here are some things that you should think about when trying to create positive relationships with your professors and teaching assistants/fellows:

- **The Name Game:** To start your relationship off, you want your teacher to know your name (at least so long as he or she learns it for a positive reason).

- **Be Organized:** Teachers are very busy people. Besides lecturing and marking exams and papers, they usually have a lot of research to do and several articles to write. When you go to see them, be organized and know exactly what it is you want to ask. Make up a list of questions that you want answered beforehand. Teachers will quickly see you as a student who does not waste their time or your own.

- **Ask Questions In Advance:** Almost all professors get annoyed by students who haven't been to their office the whole term and then bombard them with questions a few days before the exam. If you're asking fundamental questions just prior to the exam, it's quite obvious that there is no way you will ever really understand the material in time. To avoid this situation, always be up-to-date with the material you're learning. Being up-to-date means that you try to understand the course material as you move through the year. If you don't understand something, which may happen frequently, try to figure it out for yourself. However, if after a few days you still don't understand, then go see your teacher for help at that point. That way, by the time your exam arrives, you'll have had a chance to successfully integrate the material into your mind. You'll already understand it and you won't have to ask your professor basic questions that you should have been asking months earlier.

Straight A's Lesson

Build positive relationships with your professors and teaching assistants/fellows. Going to their offices with lists of questions, and asking these questions long before exams roll around, will make your teachers notice that you're a conscientious student.

Never Hesitate To Ask Questions

You are never alone at university. Whenever you have a question, however minor it may be, there are many people to turn to for answers and advice. Don't hesitate to search these people out and get the help you need. You might find yourself struggling hopelessly over something incomprehensible in a course and decide that it's your responsibility to figure it out all on your own. You're wrong! Every professor's door is open to both you and your questions.

Straight A's Lesson

Never hesitate to ask for help. Asking for help can avoid tons of frustration and save you a lot of time in the long run.

Top Ten Ways To Annoy Your Professor

- Read the newspaper in class.
- Show up to class late.
- Talk to your friends throughout class.
- Leave class early.
- Pack your books up before the end of class.
- Bombard your professor with questions immediately after class.
- Ask a question that has just been asked.
- Put your Walkman on during class.
- Sucking up – it's obvious to your professor.
- Not paying attention when your professor is answering a question that *you* asked.

Getting Reference Letters From Your Professors

Near the end of college or university you'll need to ask for reference letters from your professors when applying for jobs or graduate programs. These reference letters can be crucial. In fact, they can make or break your application.

Even if you don't know them well, most professors will write you decent reference letters if you ask for them. Your professors are not out to get you. However, it's a good idea to form a personal relationship with one or two of your professors. That way, they'll be able to offer you a more personalized, and in effect more impressive, reference letter.

When asking for reference letters, remember the following things:

- **Give the professor your resume and transcript**: The more your professor knows about you, the more detail he or she will be able to give about you in a reference letter. Make your professor's job simple by giving him or her a resume and transcript to refer to.

- **Ask in advance**: Professors are always swamped with work, and especially so when students begin asking them to write reference letters.

Asking for reference letters well in advance of needing them will ensure that your professors have plenty of time to take care in writing them.

- **Send a thank you note:** If your professor has written you a lot of reference letters, it's a good idea to show your appreciation by sending a thank you note or a small gift.

- **Make sure your professor sent your reference letter on time:** Check in once in a while to make sure that your reference letter has been sent. Professors, like anyone else, can forget to do things every now and then.

Summary

This chapter has illustrated that you're really not alone at school. There are a lot of people to meet and get to know. Start by meeting some of the people in your classes. It will make classes more enjoyable and will benefit you when you have questions or have missed a lecture. Then, try to meet some older students (students a few years ahead of you) who can give you a new perspective on classes and professors. They can also be helpful by supplying you with useful past midterm and final exams. Finally, don't forget about your professors, and perhaps more importantly, your teaching assistants and teaching fellows. You want to build positive relationships with them and avoid annoying them as much as possible. Whatever you do though, always remember: The worst mistake you can possibly make is not seeking help when you need it. There are tons of people in college to go to for advice. Make the effort to contact them.

CHAPTER 6

ORGANIZE YOURSELF FOR EXAM TIME

You're approaching your exam period at college – it's about two and a half weeks away. Terror fills the halls of your dorm or apartment. Suddenly, you frantically realize you just won't have enough time to learn all you're expected to know. However, if you've gone to class and been consistent with your note taking throughout the year as I've outlined, you can put your mind at ease. What you have to do now is pull yourself together and get organized.

Keeping yourself calm is a must during exam periods. However, it doesn't just happen by reciting a mantra every morning or increasing your exercise routine to seven days a week. You'll be confident when you have a solid plan of action in place for your exams.

It's like boarding an airplane. If you're like me and don't enjoy flying, then you probably get all uptight and nervous walking on to a plane. But the protocol established by the flight attendants and the pilots quickly puts your mind at ease. First they lock the cabin doors, then the pilot makes an announcement, and finally the safety video comes on to the screen. This procedure is familiar to you. With familiarity comes a certain level of confidence. If you entered a plane filled with commotion, that was taking off as people were standing in the aisles, and you couldn't even hear the pilot's reassuring voice, wouldn't you be a lot more nervous? I know that I would be.

Anyway, back to the point: If you have a set routine to get you organized before your exams roll around, you'll be calm and able to get down to studying with fewer distractions. This chapter deals with the three steps you have to take to get yourself ready for exam time. The **first step** is gathering all your study material into one place. You've got to organize your notes, get any notes you're missing, and rewrite your class notes so that they are more legible. The **second step** is planning that ultimate schedule that will keep you organized and focused throughout exam period. I suggest using the *Wrap Around Scheduling System* for exam time studying.

The **final step** is getting your hands on old exams. Once you get a hold of them, you've got to use them optimally. Following these three steps before you reach exam time will ease your mind and prepare you to get to work.

Prepare Your Notes For Exam Time

Let's assume you've been going to class and taking notes the way I've suggested. You've been reading your textbook and articles, and taking notes from them consistently and you've completed all your assignments for the term. It's now time to get all of these notes in order.

Organize Your Notes

You're sitting in your room and all around you are huge piles of notes in binders and files. Information is oozing off the pages. Well before you start studying for your exams, you'll need to sort through the confusion. To prepare for each exam, you'll have to divide your large volume of notes into the following piles: Class notes, textbook notes, article notes, and any assignments or exercises you've done.

Being able to locate all of your notes and having them neatly organized is a must before you hit exam time.

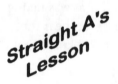

To organize yourself for exam time, gather all your notes, divide them into their respective courses, and then separate each course into individual piles of class notes, textbook notes, article notes, and assignments.

Get Any Notes You're Missing

Once you've organized your notes from each of your courses, you will be able to clearly discern which notes you are missing.

• **Class Notes:** If you've missed any classes and haven't gotten the notes from them yet, you've got to get them right away. You want to make sure that you have a complete and comprehensive set of class notes to study from for the exam.

- **Textbook Notes:** If you've been consistent with your reading and note taking from your textbooks, you should have a complete set of notes at this point. However, if you don't have a complete set, start filling in the notes that you've missed. You should then be able to put your textbook away and study only from the notes that you've taken.

- **Article Notes:** You want to ensure that you've taken notes on all the articles that you've been assigned. You also want to have on file any tutorial or class notes where these articles may have been discussed. If you feel your notes aren't complete, it's a good idea to see your professor or teaching assistant to find out what information from each article is essential to know for the exam.

- **Assignments/Exercises:** If you've had assignments or exercises to complete in a course, make sure they are all up-to-date and that your answers have all been verified and/or corrected. If you're unsure about any of your answers, go talk to a professor or teaching assistant to get them checked. You certainly don't want to be studying from wrong answers for an exam.

If you follow the above steps, you should have a complete set of notes. When you start to really study for the exam, you won't have to waste your time running around looking for the notes you're missing or trying to get answers to assignments.

Straight A's Lesson

Before exam time, get any class notes you're missing, finish any textbook and article readings you haven't done, and make sure all of your answers to class assignments are correct.

Rewrite Your Class Notes In Good Copy

I'll say it again: Your class notes are the most important data to understand for an exam. You'll need to know these notes backwards and forwards. Before you really start studying for your exam, I suggest that you copy out your class notes clearly. This might seem tedious to you at the time; however, you'll appreciate having this pristine copy of notes to study from in the long run.

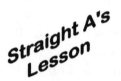 Before you even begin to study for an exam, recopy your class notes clearly.

Schedule Yourself For Exam Time

If you take a minute, close your eyes, and start to consider all of the information you must digest before you write your exam, your head might start to spin. But breaking all of this information down into sections and seeing on paper that it can be manageable will calm you down.

The Wrap Around Scheduling System

Making a study schedule is a must. But what should be your plan of attack? Here's where the *Wrap Around Scheduling System* comes in.

I'll give you a simple explanation of my *Wrap Around Scheduling System*. Let's say, for instance, that you're scheduled to write five exams. Number them in the order in which you will be writing them. In other words, exam #1 is the first one you will write and exam #5 is the last. Your plan of attack should be the reverse of what one would expect. Study first for the fifth exam, then for the fourth, the third, the second, and finally the first. Study for your last exam first and 'wrap' your way around to studying for your first exam just a few days before you're scheduled to write it.

When you get to exam period, often what happens is that you have all these exams to write and usually only a few days (or sometimes less!)

between them. Most people end up over-studying for their first two exams and then leave little or no time for their later exams. This is a self-defeating line of attack, considering that in terms of your grade point average (GPA) the last exam counts just as much as your first. What the *Wrap Around Scheduling System* emphasizes is that before you start focusing yourself on your first exam, you've got to ensure that you've significantly prepared yourself for all of the other exams that follow after it. That way, when you only have a day or two before your other exams, you'll be confident having already prepared for them. Then, all you'll have to do is concentrate on reviewing the material.

Straight A's Lesson

Use the *Wrap Around* technique to set up your study schedule. Work backwards by studying for your last exams first. This will allow you to dedicate equal time to all of your exams. Doing well means doing well on all your exams and not just on your first few.

Things To Think About When Setting Up Your Schedule

Once you find out your exam schedule, there are some things to consider before you begin to use the *Wrap Around Scheduling System*:

a) How much is the exam worth in each course?

Students generally put too much emphasis on this. When exam time rolls around, you might procrastinate by calculating what mark you'll need on each of your final exams to get an 'A'. All of my friends did it too and I too was tempted to take out my calculator and begin to calculate. However, I strongly suggest you avoid wasting your time with this nonsense.

If you decide that you want to succeed in a course, just go for it! If you do your best and follow my suggestions, you'll probably get the mark you're after. Calculating an exact number of questions you need to answer correctly to get an 'A' in a course is a complete waste of time. Instead, use that time more wisely and study. You'll probably do a lot better.

You really don't need to worry about how much each exam is worth. However, if you haven't left yourself enough time to study properly for all of your courses, you may have to ration your time. In this last scenario, the amount an exam is worth toward your final mark will become important. Obviously, you'll want to spend more time on an exam that is worth a lot more.

Straight A's Lesson

Don't waste your time figuring out what you'll need on an exam to get an 'A' as your final grade in the course. Just do your best. Follow my study suggestions and you'll get the grade you're aiming for.

b) How much time and effort will each course require?

This is the second item to consider when you arrange your study schedule for exam time. Some people believe that it all depends on the level of the course (i.e. a fourth year honors course will definitely require a lot more of your time than a first year elective). However, it doesn't always work that way. In fact, sometimes the opposite is true. Don't use the level of the course as an indication of how much time you'll need to study.

What you really want to consider when allotting time and effort for studying are the kind of questions that will be on the exam. Generally, there are three types of questions that are common to exams.

- **Memorization questions** – Many students find that these questions are the simplest type of questions found on exams. However, being able to answer them properly might require time-consuming study. Generally, studying for an exam composed mainly of pure memorization questions might not be so difficult, but it might require a lot of your time.

- **Understand and explain questions** – This second kind of question requires you to understand concepts in order to explain them properly. They are a little more difficult than pure memorization since you're not only required to memorize what you've learned, but also you must be able to understand it well enough to explain it properly. This type of exam tends to be more difficult than a pure memorization exam. However, if you've followed along consistently in a course, it might take less time to prepare for this type of exam because you'll already have the basic understanding that is necessary.

• **Applying your knowledge questions** – These are the most difficult questions to answer on any exam. First, you have to understand the material, and then you have to be able to apply what you know to new situations or problems. These really don't require that much more studying than 'understand and explain' questions do, but they might mean that you want to practice more possible test questions to ensure that you'll be able to answer whatever questions come up on your exam.

As you can see, there are three types of questions that can appear on an exam. Once you figure out what kind of questions will be on your exam, you must decide how much time and effort each of your courses will require. This depends largely on you and how you learn. If you're the type of person that understands things easily and explains them well, but it takes you a longer time to memorize information, then an 'understand and explain' exam will be a lot less time consuming for you than a pure 'memorization' exam. This is a personal aspect of your learning skills that only you can determine. There are really no set rules on how much time you should set aside to study for each exam. You have to become familiar with your learning style. This will happen by trial and error. The more exams you write, the easier it will be for you to decide how much time you need to succeed in each course.

Setting Up Your Schedule

In setting up your study schedule, you want to create a general outline that indicates when and for how long you will be studying certain subjects. Here are a few things to keep in mind when you're setting up your schedule for exam time:

Start early: Begin your study schedule for exams as soon as you can. That is, once you have all your essays and assignments out of the way for the semester, and once you have your notes organized and completed.

Overestimate the time you'll need: It is a good idea to dedicate more time to a subject than you actually anticipate you will need. Typically, people tend to underestimate how much study time will be needed for a subject. Also, things tend to come up that eliminate large chunks of the days that you originally set aside for studying. Account for these unknowns early. That way, you won't get nervous when you realize there's a lot more that you have to do in less time than you originally planned.

Divide and conquer: By dividing each course into smaller sections and then dedicating specific chunks of time to studying each section, you'll make your study goals more achievable.

Be precise: Make your schedule precise enough so that you know exactly when you should be studying each of your subjects. Seeing on paper that your schedule allows you to get everything done on time will put your mind at ease. It will also allow you to operate on 'auto-pilot' once you get into your schedule because you'll already have made the preliminary decisions as to what to study and when.

Use Past Exams

Getting your hands on past exams is a must. Your professors may make these available, they might be on reserve at the library, or you may get them from classmates, older students, or sororities or fraternities. However, just having these exams in your possession won't guarantee you an 'A' on your final exam or midterm. You've got to use them properly and know what to look for in them. I'll make this simple for you by telling you when you should be using these exams, what you should be doing with them, and how you should go about doing it.

When To Use Past Exams

As far as past exams are concerned, here's what I suggest:

- **Don't use them too early:** Some of you may try to complete past exams the minute you get your hands on them. You might think that there's no point in going over your notes now that you have the past exams in your possession. This kind of thinking is going to get you into a lot of trouble. Professors realize that students have access to these past exams and, as a result, they are highly unlikely to repeat the questions word for word on the exams they will be giving you. Therefore, studying only from these exams is not a very good idea.

• **Don't wait until the last minute**: You may decide that you'll do all of your studying first and then a day or two before the final, look at the past exams for the first time. Perhaps you think by doing this the past exams will be fresh in your memory. Unfortunately, this approach is also poorly thought out. If you wait too long to use the past exams, then you'll have very little time to get help on any questions that may arise.

• **When you should use them**: There are three points during your studies when you'll want to pick up these past exams.

• *The first round*: As soon as you get these exams in your possession, look them over right away without trying to complete them. This way, you can see the types of questions your professor prefers to ask and the information that he tends to focus upon. This preliminary information can help direct your studying.

• *The second round*: Once you recopy and have a fairly good understanding of your notes from class, you should make your first real attempt at completing these past exams.

• *The third round*: Once you've studied sufficiently for the exam, you should try again to complete the past exams.

Straight A's Lesson

There are three key times to use past exams. First, as soon as you get your hands on them, look them over to see the type of questions your professor focuses on. Second, complete the past exams in full after you've recopied your class notes. And finally, go through the past exams once more after you've sufficiently studied for your exam.

How To Use Past Exams

As we've discussed, there are three times when you should use past exams. I'll take you through each round to show you what you should be doing.

a) Your First Round At Past Exams

Look over the past exams as soon as you get them to obtain general information such as what kind of material the professor tends to test on and how he or she tends to test it.

b) Your Second Round At Past Exams

There should be a method to your madness. Here it is in three simple steps:

- **Open book exam:** When you are going through the past exams for the second round, you should be looking up the answers in your notes and not merely trying to complete them with your limited knowledge.

- **Write out your answers:** Try to get as many answers written out as possible. Just looking at the questions and deciding that you know the answers isn't going to be of much help to you. You should actually write out all the answers to help get them stored directly into your memory bank. You'll be grateful to have these answers written out for you to look over a few days before your exam.

- **Find out the answers to questions you couldn't get:** For those questions that you cannot answer, it is best to call a friend. Maybe he or she can help. However, if the two of you still can't figure it out, go see a professor.

Now you should have a fairly complete set of answers to these exam questions that you're pretty sure are accurate. It's time to go back to studying from your notes. Put away the past exams for the time being. When you have sufficiently studied for your exam, you can once again attempt the past exams for your third round.

c) Your Third Round At Past Exams

The third round of going through the past exams is a more serious one. Here is what you should be doing:

- **Simulate the real exam**: You are no longer in an open book exam – pretend it's the real thing! Close your notes and put your mind to work. On a piece of paper answer all the questions that you can. Compare these with the answers you had written down previously and that you're pretty sure are right.

- **Concentrate on the answers you got wrong**: You don't need to worry anymore about the questions you managed to answer correctly. It's time now to concentrate on those that you couldn't answer or that you got wrong. Check with your notes to see if you can figure out where you went wrong. Do you understand what your problems are? If not, talk to a classmate or a professor and see if he or she can help. However, if you do understand and you simply forgot what the correct answer was, write out that answer a few times until you're sure to remember it.

- **Strive for perfection**: By the end of your study of past exams, you should be able to answer all of the questions correctly without looking at your notes. Ignoring questions that you are not able to answer perfectly is not a clever move. You might see a question very similar to it on your upcoming exam. If you feel a need to go through the past exams a few more times before you know them adequately, do so.

Past Exams

The first round of going through past exams is merely to get an idea as to what type of questions will appear on your upcoming exam. In the second round of past exams, you want to get all the answers to the questions written out accurately and completely by looking up the answers in your notes. Then, after you have sufficiently studied for the exam, you should attempt these past exams once again in a third round. This time, test yourself by pretending it's your actual exam. See what questions you get right and which ones you get wrong and keep going over the exams (and if need be, get help) until you can answer all of the questions perfectly without looking at your notes.

Things To Look For In Past Exams

Past exams contain a lot of important information and you want to make sure that you get everything you can out of them. Here are some things to think about when you're going through past exams:

- **Types of questions your professor tends to ask**: Is the past exam made up of 'memorization', 'understand and explain', or 'apply your knowledge' questions?

- **Format of the exam**: Your professors will probably tell you ahead of time the format of your exams. If they do not, you can usually get a sense of the format from past exams. Exams that are multiple-choice will require a study tactic very different from those that are essay-based. For example, in a multiple-choice exam, you need to be able to recognize information that is correct but you need not reproduce it yourself. On the other hand, if your exam is comprised of short answer questions or longer essays, you are going to require a deeper understanding of the subject matter. This will be discussed more thoroughly at the end of Chapter Seven. However, it's important to note from the start the format of the exam that you will be writing.

- **Other possible questions**: Professors know that past exams circulate among students and they will try not to repeat questions word-for-word. At the same time, some professors find it difficult to be original and their questions from year to year will tend to resemble each other. This makes your job as a student simple. You have to make logical predictions of the questions your professor will be likely to ask on your exam. This might seem hard to you in the beginning, but after some practice you'll see a pattern and be able to make educated guesses as to questions that might appear on your upcoming exams. By my third and fourth year at university, I was able to accurately predict exam questions. This certainly wasn't a sign of genius in me. All I did was carefully look over past exams, and the information that we studied in class, and made logical guesses as to what would appear on the upcoming exam. If you have some knowledge about what the questions will be on an exam, you can ensure that you'll be able to answer them expertly by properly preparing for them beforehand.

Straight A's Lesson

Work through past exams thoroughly and make sure you can answer all questions correctly. Then, step back and evaluate what types of questions your professor tends to ask, what the format of the exam will be, and try to predict the questions that will appear on your upcoming exam.

Summary

There you have it! You now know what you have to do to prepare yourself properly for exam time. You've got to get organized, and the first step toward getting organized relates to your notes. Sort them out, track down any that you're missing, and then rewrite them in good. The next thing to think about is creating a schedule for exam time. You want to study for your last exam first, and then 'wrap around' to studying for your first exam using the *Wrap Around Scheduling System*. When making your schedule, you want to consider how much time and effort each course will require. You can rework and adjust your schedule as needed, but it's important that you have one to start out with. Finally, you want to get your hands on past exams. Once you get them, you should keep going over them until you can answer all of the questions perfectly without looking at your notes. If you do all of these things, you'll be ready to get down to serious studying. See the next chapter for my introduction to the ICE method of study.

CHAPTER 7

USE A STUDY METHOD

To be honest, I really had no idea what I was doing during my first year of university. When exam time came, I felt submerged under large piles of notes and I ended up wasting a lot of time just trying to figure out what to do. With some expert advice from my family members whom had all gone through the same frenzied situation, I came up with a solid, reliable, and simple method of study. This method has kept me calm during exams, and consistently brought me the straight A's I've been looking for. Thinking back, I can give this method credit for my acceptance into an Ivy League graduate program.

The first thing I'll do in this chapter is present an overview of the importance of using a study method. Then, I'll discuss the method of my choice, which I call the ICE method (Issue Condensation for Exam Method). I'll show you exactly what it is and give you all the information you'll need to understand how to apply it. Finally, you'll need a battery of tricks that will help you with your studying. They include making lists, using acronyms, and unloading your information when you begin your exam. I'll discuss them in depth at the end of the chapter.

Overview Of A Study Method

You'll probably take four to five courses a semester and have to write a few exams as well. A lot of stress is inevitable. However, having a study method can really help.

The Importance Of A Study Method

There are three good reasons why you should have a study method:

- **Studying becomes a routine**: When you have a solid study method, studying starts to become routine. As a result, studying gets easier and easier simply because you're getting used to it.

- **You avoid useless dilemmas**: A study method helps you avoid dilemmas about how to study. Figuring out how to study for each course is a task in itself. You sit down to a huge pile of notes overflowing with information from your classes, textbook, articles, and assignments, but you just don't know where to begin. However, if you have a study method, your dilemmas will dissipate into thin air. You'll know exactly what to do and when to do it and you won't need to waste your time deliberating about it.

- **It builds up your confidence**: If you stick to a study method and you discover it works for you time after time, you build up confidence in your ability to do well. Having this confidence will quell your fears about upcoming exams. Avoiding useless anxiety during exam periods will make you feel better, sleep more deeply, and think more clearly.

Straight A's Lesson

Having a study method is essential in school. It makes studying become routine, helps you avoid dilemmas over how you should be studying, and gives you confidence in your ability to do well.

Characteristics Of A Good Study Method

Now that we've established the importance of having a study method, we've got to think about what makes a method successful. There are three important criteria that a good method needs to satisfy. Your method of studying should be:

- **Effective**: This means that when you religiously adhere to this method, you should get the grades you're aiming for.

- **Efficient**: Using your method should mean that you are not wasting your time studying things that are unimportant. Your study method should allow you to get the most useful studying done in the least amount of time possible.

- **Applicable over a wide range of subjects.** In order for a study method to become routine, you must be able to apply the same method to almost all of your courses. Being able to use your method only for an English course is not enough. The method you use must be applicable to all subjects, from microbiology to philosophy and everything in between.

Straight A's Lesson   **When you choose a study method, make sure that it works, that it is efficient, and that it can be used for most of your courses.**

Chose A Method And Stick To It

Once you discover a method that works for you, you've got to stick to it. You can't just say, "Oh, it's too tiresome and boring!" Once a method does become routine, it probably will get a little boring. That's the beauty of it! We're trying to make studying for exams almost as simple and straightforward as tying your shoes. It will not work if you give up too easily however.

Be dedicated to a study method. As long as it gets you the grades that you're aiming for, overlook the fact that it can get a little tedious. After all, studying in general is a tedious exercise.

Straight A's Lesson   **You really have to stick to a study method even if you feel that it's boring. As long as it works for you, continue with it and you'll have it mastered by the end of your school career.**

The ICE Method (Issue Condensation for Exam Method)

Now that we're past the preliminary stuff, we can get to the core of this section. Here I'll present my own reliable method of study. It has helped me succeed in all of my undergraduate courses and it helped me get into the graduate program I desired. With a little dedication, it can do the same for you.

Steps To The ICE Method

The ICE Method is a method of studying for exams. It stands for the Issue Condensation Method for Exams.

We've already gone over how to take notes during the year and how to get you prepared for exam time.

When it gets to within a few weeks before your exams, you should be left with a complete set of *legible* and *organized* notes. You shouldn't need to look back at your messy class notes, since you've gone to the trouble of writing them out in full and legible form. You also shouldn't have to refer to your textbook or articles anymore as you've already taken notes on them. Now it's time to start studying according to the ICE Method. Here's what you should do:

Step 1: Class Notes

You should begin with your class notes. Class notes, as we discussed in Chapter Three, are almost always the most important sources of information to know for exams. You already have a recopied, neat set of notes from your class. Now you're going to copy them out again, but this time you want to focus on *condensing* them using the following guidelines:

- **Get Organized**: Sometimes, a professor will talk about a certain topic in one class and then continue with it a few lectures later as a review. You want to bring together all of the information relating to a certain topic for your new set of notes. What you're trying to do is reorganize your notes into logical and coherent sections. This will allow you to recognize all the repetition that appears in your notes.

- **Eliminate Repetition**: Professors love to repeat themselves! But, you won't love rewriting the same line in your notes over and over again. Therefore, you should condense what your professor has said by eliminating the repetition in your notes. However, you should, at the same time, take notice of what information was repeated by the professor - it's usually what he or she considers centrally important and what will most likely show up on one of your exams.

- **Be Neat**: Your goal is to condense your notes. Writing more neatly and in smaller print will leave you with a shorter set of notes to study from.

- **Simplify Information**: Try to simplify information by taking out useless words and getting to the core of the idea. This will reduce the number of words you write down.

- **Go Slow To Understand**: The most important thing to do when you're condensing your notes for the first time is to go slow in order to understand the material. Go through each step in your professor's train of thought in order to figure out the logic behind what they have said. If you're having problems, don't worry! There are a lot of people you can approach for help. It's a good idea to put tabs in places that are problematic. Then, when you've gathered up a few questions, you can ask a classmate or a professor about them all at once.

- **Struggle With The Information**: Before you do go to seek help, try to figure out the material on your own. Struggling with your notes is worthwhile because if you do end up figuring out the problematic areas on your own, you'll gain confidence. Moreover, you will have learned the material more thoroughly.

Straight A's Lesson

The first step in the ICE Method is making a fresh set of class notes to study from. While you are recopying your notes, try to condense them by reorganizing them, eliminating repetition, writing neatly, and simplifying the information. You will end up with a much shorter set of notes than you started out with.

Step 2: Condense Further

Now you're going to recopy your notes again. Using the same techniques, you want to make your new set of notes significantly shorter than the previous set. This will happen quite naturally without your even thinking about it. How? Well, when you go through your notes to condense them for a second time, you'll find that you have an automatic instinct as to what words and information you should be writing down and what you should be leaving out. You'll be so much more familiar with the information that, as a result, you'll end up only writing about half as much as you wrote down in the earlier set of notes.

At the end of Step 2, you should have a much shorter set of notes to study from. You'll be able to breathe a big sigh of relief when you discover that there isn't really as much information as you had anticipated. That's the best part of the condensation method. It makes you realize that studying for your upcoming exam isn't nearly as difficult as you thought it might be. This is the advantage of condensing your material.

Step 3: Condense Further

Believe it or not, you're now going to condense your notes even further still. You might start to think that this is getting really boring. Sorry to burst your bubble! That's what happens when you have a set routine for doing something – it does become boring. As boring as you might think it is at the time however, you won't complain when you realize the night before your exam, that, unlike your friends who are scrambling through their unorganized and unmethodical notes, you are completely relaxed and raring to go. You'll be happier still when you get your exam back with one of the highest grades in your class.

As you can see, the point of this method is to keep condensing and condensing. You should continue to do this until your notes take up just a few sheets of paper. My father often brags that when he went to law school, he could fit the notes of a full-year course on to a piece of paper the size of his palm. I was never able to condense my notes that small, but the method has still worked amazingly well for me. Don't sweat it! Getting your class notes down to a few pages is good enough.

Continue to condense your notes until you think that they have reached their minimum length and then proceed to the final step.

Final Step: Test Yourself

It's time to prove to yourself that you really do know all of the information that you've been recopying. You do this by testing yourself. This will let you see exactly what you know and what you don't. Go through your notes and prepare questions for yourself based on all of the information that appears in your last set of notes. Then, try to answer these questions without looking at your notes.

You'll be surprised to see that when you write out your answers to the questions you've come up with, you'll be writing down a whole lot more than you had actually written out in your final set of condensed notes. This is exactly what is supposed to happen. When you are answering a question, your brain will automatically start expanding the information that you have condensed. In effect, you'll write an answer that includes a lot of the information that you filtered away during the condensation process.

This happens naturally and is the point of the study method. I call it the **domino effect**. Each word that you write down in your final set of notes triggers your mind to recall more and more of the information related to the topic. One short word can make you think of something else, which will make you think of something else, etc. Your professor marking the exam will be utterly impressed with your ability to retain so much information. The irony of it all is that you didn't even think that you retained this much information, considering how short your study notes were.

When you are testing yourself, you should take note of the questions (if any) you had trouble with. Then, you should go back and see where you went wrong. If you didn't understand the material, get some help. If you did understand the material but you had just forgotten it, take some time to write it out a couple of times. This will help you to learn it and remember it for the real exam.

Keep testing yourself until you can answer all the questions you've prepared for yourself to the best of your ability. Now you're prepared for any exam, however difficult it may be.

The morning before your exam, merely read over your last set of condensed notes. By then, you'll feel comfortable and ready to ace it.

The ICE Method

The ICE Method is all about recopying and condensing your notes. You do this until you have a short set of notes to study from for your exam, usually a few pages in length. The final thing to do is to test yourself on information that you should know. Play this game over and over again until you know everything you need to know for the exam. Finally, the morning before the exam, look over your final set of notes so that the information is fresh in your mind.

I've focused on dealing with class notes to highlight the ICE method, but what are you supposed to do with the rest of the information that you must know for an exam such as textbook and article material? I'll tell you in three simple words: Condense, combine, and conquer.

- **Condense:** You want to use the same method that you used for your class notes to condense your textbook and article notes. You should end up with a short set of notes from these sources.

- **Combine:** The next step is to try to combine the information from your textbook and articles with your class notes by finding the sections that overlap. That way, you will end up with just one complete set of notes to study from.

- **Conquer:** Now that you have all of your notes combined, you can conquer the information all at once. By now, you should have your notes condensed to a mere few pages. Test yourself to see what you do and don't know.

Why This Method Works So Well

You probably are wondering why this method works so well. How does it allow you to retain such a large portion of the information you're studying? Here are three reasons why this method works the wonders that it does:

- **It's an active method**: The ICE Method forces you to be actively involved in your studying. Writing out your notes over and over again as you condense them to make them shorter and shorter, is a physical job. You can't possibly lose your focus because you are actively doing something. Other methods of studying, such as reading your notes over and over again while reciting them, are much more passive. They aren't as effective because your head begins to wander and you start to daydream.

- **It brings out the main issues**: By forcing you to condense your notes, the ICE Method ends up directing you to the core of what you should be studying. You'll sort through the extraneous material and come to the summary points (see Chapter 4) of the subject matter. You'll really get the point that your professor has been trying to make.

- **The domino effect**: I've mentioned this effect already, but it is important to reiterate it. As you condense your notes, your notes get shorter and shorter and you end up with a few key words on your final summary sheets that trigger your mind to think of all the information that you've filtered away. That way, even though you feel you're only learning a small amount of material (and you're appreciative that it's a manageable amount to study), when you actually write your exam, you are able to expand the ideas into a much larger and more comprehensive explanation because of the trigger effect.

Why I personally love this method

My intention in my study plan is to be as efficient as I can be. If I am going to be stuck in the library studying for a day, I don't want to waste my time reading over my notes if they won't stick in my head. When I rewrite my notes to condense them, I not only learn and retain my notes, but I also finish with a superlative set of new notes to refer to and study from. This new set of notes is always shorter than the last and as a result, I become more and more efficient. It never feels like I've learned that much information because I get everything down to just a few sheets. But, boy – on the day of the exam, I realize that I know a lot!

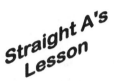

The ICE Method works so well because it's an active method, because it makes you get to the core point of the subject matter, and because of the domino effect. The time you spend studying is used as efficiently as possible.

The ICE Method Satisfies The Criteria For A Good Study Method

Let's go back to our criteria for a "good method" we outlined earlier in this chapter and see if the ICE Method qualifies as one:

- Does it work? It works for me and for anyone I've suggested it to. I'm certain it will work for you to.

- It's efficient: Actively learning your material is the best way to ensure that you're making the most of your study time.

- It's applicable over a wide range of courses: Nothing in this method is specific to any course or subject. It can be used in everything from math, economics, or chemistry classes to English or philosophy courses.

Straight A's Lesson

The ICE Method satisfies the criteria for a good method since it works, it's efficient, and it's applicable over a wide range of courses.

Other Important Tricks To Studying

Employing a study method will definitely help you get the A's you're aiming for. But, you should also know about some of the other tricks to studying. These can really help you when it comes down to crunch time.

Make Lists And Number The Items On The Lists

In front of you is all of this information. To learn the material, it certainly is helpful to put it in some kind of order. One way to do this is by putting the material that you've learned into lists. For example, while discussing the cinematic devices used in *Citizen Kane*, the professor might go on for about a half an hour. In your notes, you have all of the information about all of the different cinematic devices that you're going to have to know for the final exam. To make it easier to study them, you want to make a list of the different cinematic devices.

Once you've made your list of information points, give them each a number. This will make it much easier for you to remember how many cinematic devices there are in Citizen Kane and to recall each of them.

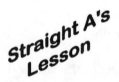 **If you've got a lot of information to know about a certain topic, turn the information into a list and number the articles in that list. This will make the information easier for you to recall in an exam.**

Acronyms

Once you've made up these lists and numbered each item, a great way to help you recall the information in its entirety is to use acronyms. Here's how to use acronyms:

- Pick out a key word from each article in the list.
- Write down the first letter of each key word.
- You'll be left with a bunch of random letters to remember.
- Make up a little phrase or catchy saying that will help you recall all of the letters.

As long as you remember the phrase at the exam, you'll have the first letter of each article on the list. Then, you'll be able to work backwards and recall all of the information on the list.

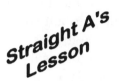

Use acronyms to help you remember information that you've put in lists. Think up catchy phrases that will be easy for you to recall at an exam.

Unload Your Information

This is an important trick that you should use once you get into your exam. You'll probably have a bunch of acronyms memorized, as well as formulas and other important information. As soon as you're allowed to begin, unload all of this information on to the front sheet of your exam. That way, your mind can relax since you no longer have to carry around the memorized information in your head.

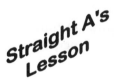

As soon as you get into the exam, unload information that you've been memorizing such as lists, acronyms, or formulas.

In the Exam

When you're in the exam, there are certain things you should be doing and thinking about to maximize your grade. Here's what I suggest:

- **Make sure you have all the pages of an exam**: When you first turn over your exam, you'll see on the cover that it indicates how many pages should be there. Quickly make sure that you have everything that you're supposed to.

- **Watch the clock**: In any exam, there is a time limit. Running out of time is something you want to avoid, especially if the last question on the exam is the easiest (or worth the most marks). At the beginning of the exam, quickly calculate how much time you should devote to each section based on the amount each question is worth. This will give you a time frame to work with during your exam.

- **Do the easy questions first**: It's a good idea to do the easy questions on the exam first, for two reasons. First, there's always the possibility that you might run out of time and you wouldn't want to leave any easy questions unanswered. Second, doing the easier questions first will boost your confidence, allowing you to soar through the rest of the exam. So, when you first look at the exam, survey the different questions, determine which questions are easiest, and begin with these.

- **Don't get stuck**: The worst thing you can do on an exam is get stuck on a question. If you come across a question that you're having a lot of trouble with, go on with the rest of the exam and come back to it at the end. Otherwise, you'll waste too much time on that question (and you may not even get it right!) and you won't have enough time to finish your exam.

- **Check over your answers**: Always make sure to leave enough time at the end of your exam to check over your answers. This will give you a chance to correct potential mistakes such as the following: reading a question wrong, skipping over a question, or forgetting to include an important point in an answer.

- **Give more attention to questions with more weight**: You should be aware that some questions are worth more than others. A question worth fifty points will require a lot more attention and effort than a question on the same exam worth only fifteen. In addition, you must realize that your professor is expecting a lot in an answer that's worth a large portion of your exam. So, even if a question sounds simple, if it's worth 50% of your grade on your final exam, you should write out a fairly in-depth answer.

- **Verify you've answered all the questions**: You'll kick yourself if you get your exam back and realize that you absent-mindedly skipped over a whole section. To avoid this, get into the habit of verifying that you've answered everything on your exam before you hand it in. A good way to do this is by adding up all the possible marks for each question and making sure that it equals the total amount of possible marks on the entire exam.

- **Ask questions whenever you have them**: Usually, your professor will be at the exam. If you have any questions, however trivial you might think they may be, ask them. A lot of times, it may be hard for you to understand what exactly the professor wants. Don't ever guess at the professor's intentions. Ask him or her directly. While your professor answers your query during an exam, your professor might even hint at whether or not you're on the right track with your answer. If for some reason your professor is not present during the exam, write down any questions you have on the front cover. If there is a problem with your mark after the exam, you'll have proof that you had thought the question was ambiguous to begin with.

Multiple-Choice Exams

In a multiple-choice question, there is usually a stem followed by four or five possible answers. Here is an example:

The best way to study for an exam, according to the book *Ten Ways to Straight A's* is:

- Reciting information over and over again.
- Reading your notes.
- Studying in groups.
- Using the Issue Condensation Method for Exams.

If you've paid attention, you'll know the answer is (d). At any rate, in this example, the stem of the question is: "The best way to study for an exam, according to the book *Ten Ways To Straight A's* is ...". The items listed under the stem are the selection of possible answers. Your job on multiple-choice questions is to choose one, and only one, of the possible answer choices given.

Here are some things you should remember when taking multiple-choice tests and exams:

- **Your first answer is usually the right one**: The majority of times, when you change your answer on a multiple-choice exam, you're changing the right answer to a wrong one. Therefore, unless you really know that you're changing your answer to the correct one, learn to trust your first instinct.

- **Hide the answers when reading the stem**: When I do multiple-choice questions, I read the stem first without looking at the choices listed. I try to fill in the sentence or answer the question myself. Only then do I peak at the choices given. This gives me an advantage when I look through the possible choices since I already have a strong sense of what I'm looking for.

- **Elimination is the key**: If you're not positive which is the correct answer, it's a good idea to eliminate the answers that you know are wrong for certain. Cross them out right on the exam paper then concentrate on the answers that remain. If you have to guess between the answers that remain, realize that you've significantly increased your chances at being correct by eliminating some wrong answers.

- **Exaggerations**: If one of your answer choices contains any of the following words in the text, there is a good chance that it's incorrect: 'Any', 'all', 'everybody', 'everything', or 'everywhere'. From my experience, if a choice appears to make a sweeping generalization, it is usually not the correct one.

- **Read the stem of the question carefully**: There are some key words that you should underline in the stem that indicate what type of answer you are looking for. For example, the stem might say, "Which one of the following four statements is not correct …". Make sure you underline the word 'not' in the stem. In this question, you want to eliminate those answer choices that you know are true. The wording in the stem will determine what kind of answer you'll be looking for. So, read the stem over a few times to make sure you understand what's being asked.

- **See the exam as one unit**: In long multiple-choice exams, there will be a few questions relating to the same topic. In this case, if you can't get an answer to a certain question, look to see if there are any other questions in the exam that deal with the same topic. A similar question might help you figure out what the correct answer is for the question that is troubling you.

- **Keep moving along**: If you don't know the answer to a question right away, circle it and come back to it at the end. You never want to get bogged down on any exam, especially a multiple-choice one. You might be surprised to discover that when you come back to the same question later on, it doesn't seem as difficult as you had previously thought.

- **Marking the answer on the scan card**: In most multiple-choice exams, you'll have to bubble in your answers on a scan card. Be careful that you've bubbled in the correct answer. It's easy to screw up when you transfer your answer from the exam paper to the scan card. I suggest that once you've gone through your exam, go through it one final time to double-check your answers and to make sure you've bubbled in the correct spot. Here are some other things to think about when you're using scan cards:

  - Make sure you've bubbled in the correct version number of your exam on your scan card.
  - Use a dark (HB) pencil.
  - Erase any wrong answers completely.
  - Erase any markings at the sides of your paper that might interfere with the computer's analysis of your scan card.

Open Book Exams

Your professor tells you that you'll be able to bring in all of your notes to your final exam. You're thrilled! You were planning to study for hours and hours for the exam, but now you *think* you're off the hook. Think again!

Open book exams are a little bit of a trick. Your professor will usually give you an open book exam when either:

- He or she knows that you won't have time to look at your notes during the exam because you'll be under such a huge time constraint.

Or

- Your professor knows your notes will be useless since most of the questions will be "applying your knowledge" questions (see Chapter 6).

So, an open book exam is not worthy of a celebration. However, there are ways to do well on these exams as long as you realize that you're not off the hook for studying. Here's what you have to do:

- **Follow the ICE Method**: You still need to prepare yourself as much as you can for this exam, especially since open book exams are often the most difficult.

- **Be organized**: You want your notes to be as organized as possible so that if you have to look something up during your exam, you'll be able to find it right away. A good idea is to use Post-it™ notes. They'll help you retrieve the information you're looking for as quickly as you can.

- **Past exams**: You should have all of the answers to these at your fingertips. If you see a question on your exam that looks familiar to you, you can double check your answer with the one you've written out when going over past exams.

- **Apply-your-knowledge questions**: Usually your professor will give you an open book exam when most of the questions on the exam will be "apply- your-knowledge questions" (see Chapter 6). You've got to really understand the information that you've learned and be able to apply that knowledge to other questions/situations. You should be going through practice questions when studying for the exam (i.e. by doing old exams, assignments, and exercises) rather than bothering to memorize information. You have your notes there if you need to look up anything.

- **Make a quick reference sheet**: You want to make sure that you have a sheet handy full of important information. You'll probably be using it to refer to throughout your exam.

Take Home Exams

Occasionally, you'll be assigned a take home exam. It can be one of several different types. Regardless, make sure that you remember the following:

- **Prepare in advance**: Do any readings or assignments that you need to do in preparation for your exam. You might be under a time constraint.

- **Strive for perfection**: Writing a take home exam is not like writing an in-class exam at all. Since you have much more time to complete a take home exam, professors expect much higher quality from you. Professors will expect a minimum of mistakes in a take home exam. You should aim to satisfy this criterion. If you're writing an essay, make sure that it's edited to death (see essay writing, Chapter 9). If you're completing a math or science assignment, avoid any silly calculation errors. Whatever the case, check over your take home exam thoroughly and, if possible, get someone else to look it over to make sure you're handing in a high quality exam.

- **Compare with others**: Never copy a take home exam from someone else. Professors and teaching assistants/fellows look them over very carefully and can often discover who has merely copied someone else's exam. It could mean a zero on your exam, so avoid doing this. However, it's a good idea to compare your answers with someone else to see if you're on the right track. If you've both arrived at similar answers, then you've most likely completed your assignment correctly.

- **Plan ahead and leave yourself time:** If you know that you'll be assigned a take home exam on a certain date, then make sure when you get it that you'll be able to dedicate a large portion of your time to it until it's done. Plan ahead and complete all the other work that you'll have to do during that time period. That way, when you get the take home exam, you'll be able to devote 100 percent of your attention to it.

Answering Essay Questions On Exams

You might have an exam in a political science or history course that is primarily composed of questions requiring you to write out long answers. Do these exams correctly by following this advice:

- **Write neatly**: If your professors can't read what you've written then they can't mark it properly. Try to write as neatly as you can. You'll make the marker's job easier and he or she will appreciate it. Hopefully your mark will reflect this appreciation.

- **Stick to the point**: It's very easy in a written answer to include a lot of information that doesn't really answer the question. This tends to annoy the person who is marking the exam and gives him or her the impression that you're just trying to fill up space and that you really don't know the answer to the question being asked. Try and stick to answering the question at hand in written exams.

- **Write an outline**: Whenever you have to write essays on an exam, always write an outline for your essay before you begin it. Plan out what you want to say in each paragraph and make sure that the essay you've planned will answer the question posed. Only then should you start to write. If you make an outline first, your essay will be organized and focused on the question that is being asked.

- **Don't waste time**: In any written exam, you'll likely have a lot to write down in a short amount of time. Make the most of your time! Don't waste precious moments by thinking about a question for too long. If you've studied the material as I've outlined in this chapter, you should have no problem quickly coming up with an outline and getting to work on writing out your answer in full. This will ensure that you have enough time to complete the entire exam.

- **Massage your hand**: When you stop to think about what you're going to write for the next question on your exam, stretch out your hand and massage it briefly to avoid it getting cramped up.

- **Energy bursts**: Personally, I find written exams to be very tiring. I always bring some candies with me and whenever I start to feel exhausted, I pop one into my mouth for a quick burst of energy.

- **Show your knowledge**: Think of written exams as a time to show how much you've been studying and how well you've retained the information. It's one thing to know a lot, but it won't help out your grade much if your professor isn't aware of what you know. When answering a question, be as thorough as possible. Include all information that is pertinent.

- **Don't get caught up with writing style**: Exams are one of the only times when you really don't need to be worrying about your writing style (unless, of course, you're an English major). For the most part, professors are looking more at content in written exams and are less concerned with how you present the information.

- **Read directions carefully**: It's crucial that you read the instructions on written exams carefully. You want to look for words such as *compare*, *contrast*, *illustrate*, and *define* to ensure that you're giving the professor what he or she is looking for.

Getting Back An Exam

Whenever you get an exam back, you should look it over to determine if the mark has been properly assigned:

- Make sure the professor added up your mark correctly.
- Look to see what questions you got wrong.
- Decide whether you're satisfied with your professor's marking of the exam.

If you have found a mathematical error in your grade, talk to the professor immediately. Your professor will probably have no problem changing your grade as long as you point out the mistake right away.

If there is no mathematical error, but you still think that you deserve a higher grade on the exam, determine why you think you deserve one. Go through the questions that you got wrong and articulate on a piece of paper why you 'should have' received a higher mark. Take this list to your professor and calmly discuss your mark. If you really do deserve a higher mark and you are rational in your reasoning, your professor might listen to you and change your grade.

If your professor is adamant that your grade should remain as it is, there are a few possible tactics you can then resort to:

- If you still think you deserve a higher grade (and you're pretty sure that a different professor would feel the same way) you can appeal your grade to a higher authority. Go talk to your faculty administrators to find out the process to appeal a mark on an exam.

- If you're not that sure that you deserve a higher grade and don't want to go through the appeal process, then decide to leave the mark as it is. Doing this will ensure that you avoid annoying your professor. Instead, it's a good idea to talk to your professor about how you can improve to get the grade you want on your next exam.

Whatever you decide to do about a grade that you are not happy with, go about it rationally. You will never get a mark changed on an exam if you're overly emotional about it. However, if your reason through your argument logically, and your professor can see that, you'll have a much better chance of seeing a change made in your grade.

Summary

After reading this chapter, you should have a good idea of how to study for your exams. I've emphasized that in order to do well you really need a study method to guide you. I've presented my personal favorite, the ICE Method. It works, it's efficient, and it's applicable over a wide range of courses. I suggest you adopt this method as soon as possible and stick with it. If you do, your marks will soar and so will your confidence. Finally, I've given you a few other tips to think about when you're studying. Lists and acronyms are simple devices that will make learning chunks of information much simpler. And, when you get to the exam, don't forget to quickly write down all of your memorized data on to the first page. Now that you're on your way to developing a reliable study routine, I'll let you in on some other things you should know that will help you get through exam time with your nerves intact.

CHAPTER 8

SURVIVE EXAM TIME

If you're like many of the people I know, you probably find that exam time is not a walk in the park. In fact, prior to exams you might have trouble sleeping, experience terrible headaches, or suffer from painful stomachaches. Even if you don't get any of these symptoms, you might just find yourself obsessively counting down the days until your exams are over.

Yes, exam time can be a pain in the neck. Who wouldn't rather be relaxing, shopping, or doing anything else for that matter? The fact is, however, that you've got to get through exam time because it's an integral part of almost any university or college program. I want to help you get through it in the best possible way.

The first thing I'll discuss in this chapter is how to remain calm during exam time. I give you suggestions on how to keep your cool and assure you that some stress during exam time can actually be beneficial. Next, I'll discuss the importance of getting into a routine which includes going to bed at a reasonable time every night, having fun on the weekends, and giving yourself study breaks during your long, tiring days. Finally, I'll give you the scoop on where and with whom to study. By using these techniques, you should be able to survive exam time without any major distresses.

Keep Calm

When I get frazzled, I'm unable to think properly. Under the same circumstances, you probably can't think your best either. Yet, exam time is certainly one time when you definitely want to think clearly. That's why you have to make every effort to keep calm, cool, and collected. Let me give you some tips on what you should and shouldn't be doing.

Get Stressed Out Early

Inevitably, exam time causes stress. In fact, I too feel stress during exam time. However, I have found a way to help me get through exams. I suggest you give this method a try. I begin to think about my exams a few weeks ahead of time. At that time I get organized, rewrite my notes, and start scheduling myself. Because I begin exam preparations early, I also get stressed out early - early enough to get over it in time.

I plan far enough in advance so that I can see that I'll be able to accomplish all I set out to. By stressing out early, when it comes to crunch time (a few days before all of my exams are starting), I feel considerably calmer.

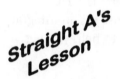

Get stressed out a few weeks *before* **exam time (if you're going to at all). That way, by the time you get to exam period, you'll be a lot more relaxed and focused.**

Relax The Night Before The Exam – Review Your Notes In The Morning

You may pick up on a certain routine that is typical for many university students: Staying up all night before an exam and cramming. Do yourself a favor and forget about testing this method out.

You'll need a good night's sleep before your exam. After all, it's when we're sleeping that our minds mull over information we've learned and make sense of it all. Needless to say, cramming doesn't provide you with this necessary interlude. Besides, do you really think you'll be alert on the day of the exam if you've been up the whole night before?

If you have planned your studying carefully, there should be little left for you to do the night before the exam. I would usually finish studying early, and then take time out to relax, either by watching some mindless TV or by talking on the phone. Taking a little time the night before an exam just to cool off can be very helpful. In addition, you'll find that if you stop studying early and do something relaxing, it will be easier to fall asleep. Getting a solid night's sleep is essential before a long exam.

So try to relax a little the night before your exam. That's not to say that you should go out drinking and come home at four o'clock in the morning. However, you should take some time out just to loosen up.

Relaxing the night before an exam is a good idea. But, what should you do on the morning of the exam? As a rule, I always wake up early the morning of my exams in order to review course material. I also test myself on formulas, acronyms, and any lists that I have to remember. That way, all of the information is fresh in my head when I walk into the exam and I'm ready and eager to show what I know.

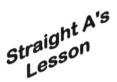

If you've scheduled yourself well, you should have little to do the night before an exam. That way, you can take some time out for yourself and relax. In the morning, you should wake up early and review the material, making sure that you remember anything you've memorized, such as formulas.

A Little Bit of Stress Is Actually A Good Thing

Your teeth chatter as you walk into your exam. Your hand is shaking so much that you're handwriting resembles your baby brother's. Too much stress is never a good thing, especially when it tends to block your ability to think clearly. Still, feeling absolutely no stress at all is not a good thing either.

When I began university, I'd get quite nervous walking into an exam. Butterflies would flit around in my stomach and I'd feel all fidgety inside. My mother would attempt to console me by assuring me that having a little stress could actually work to my benefit when I walk into an exam. "A little stress will keep you alert," she'd say.

Let me give you an analogy to help you understand this point more clearly. Imagine yourself walking down a dark alley when, out of the corner of your eye, you notice someone following close behind you. It looks like he's going to rob you and you're terrified! So, you run away more quickly than you ever thought possible.

Similarly, when you walk into an exam, it's not such a good idea to be so calm that your pulse has practically stopped. A little bit of stress can help you perform beyond your usual limitations.

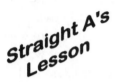

A little bit of stress can be beneficial in an exam. It will increase your adrenalin and allow you to perform better than you thought possible.

Get Into A Routine During Exam Time

During exam time, there's so much to get done and so little time to do it. Still, you've got to sleep, eat, and do everything else you can to stay healthy, both in mind and body. As well, you've got to take time out to relax, go out with friends, and have some fun to keep sane and somewhat happy during exam time.

No Late Nights Studying

You're going to have a lot of work to get done during exam time (and the entire school year for that matter). You must get into a routine that can sustain you over the long term. Staying up until four in the morning isn't a routine you'll be able to keep up, especially when you have to wake up for nine o'clock exams.

Personally, I preferred getting an early start on my studying. I would wake up at eight thirty, and start studying by nine or nine thirty. But, no matter how much work I did that day, I would stop studying at a reasonable time, usually around ten o'clock at night. I called it the **ten o'clock rule**.

Since I would stop studying at ten o'clock, I had a chance to relax for a while before going to bed. Getting into this kind of routine allowed me to consistently get up early in the morning, put in a good day of studying, and go to bed at a reasonable time. In addition, early exams were not a problem since I was used to waking up at that time and my mind was accustomed to being alert and fresh early in the morning.

Straight A's Lesson

Try not to stay up too late during exam time. Get into the habit of finishing your studying around ten o'clock. That way, you'll be able to get a good night's sleep and be awake early the next morning.

Make Sure You Still Have Some Fun

Exam time, and your whole year for that matter, can be very depressing if you never take time out for fun. Remember to let your hair down and relax every now and then.

Regardless of how much work I had to do during exam time, I always took Friday and Saturday nights off. This kept me sane during exam period. A movie and a dinner with friends can revitalize your energy.

Straight A's Lesson

Make sure you still have some fun during your exams. It will keep your spirits up and will make you more able to focus on your studies.

Include Study Breaks Every Two Hours

Let's say you go to the library to immerse yourself in your books for the day. You're sitting at your cubicle condensing your notes over and over again and your hand starts to ache. Then, your eyes start to close. You know you're not going to be very productive at this point.

To avoid useless studying (i.e. studying when you're unable to concentrate) you want to make sure that you routinely take breaks. Every 1 ½ to 2 hours you should make sure to get up from your seat and take some time out from your work. It may mean going to the cafeteria to grab a coffee or a snack, or taking a short walk around campus. Whatever works for you is best. The point is, remember to stretch your legs and give your mind a chance to rest.

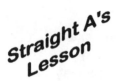

Two hours of study is about all that your mind can handle in one sitting so make sure that you give yourself breaks.

The Scoop On Where To Study

Similar to finding your favorite seat in each of your classes, you should be able to find a place to study where you can concentrate and be comfortable. In this section I give you some things to think about when deciding where to study.

Library Evaluation

Throughout the regular school year, you might like going to the main library in between classes or on the weekend to get a lot of work done. You might find it to be a super-quiet hideaway from the constant distractions of the telephone, TV, and refrigerator at home.

However, at exam time, the tranquility in the main library will fade and soon disappear altogether. Suddenly, the quiet hideaway you're used to is brimming with students. Everywhere you look you see your friends, classmates, and people you know. What's normally a nice, quiet atmosphere becomes a happening social scene. It might be fun for a while, but soon you'll get an uneasy feeling as you remember that exam time is fast approaching. Your nerves are shot, and you're ready to scream at the next person who annoys you. This might be a good time for you to find another place to study.

It's a good idea during exam time to find a library that is not as well known to people, especially by those you know. When I was in university, at exam time I studied in the Law Library instead of at the main library on campus. It was quieter and more relaxing since I didn't know many people there.

Before you plunk down and claim your study space, venture out to different libraries. You might discover that some libraries are more conducive to studying than the main library you're used to.

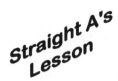 If the main library is too distracting during exam time, try out other smaller libraries that aren't as popular.

The Right Kind Of People To Study With

There are certain people you want to surround yourself with during exam time and there are those you should avoid all together. Here is my advice:

- **Friends:** Studying with friends is fine if your friends are considerate and won't try to distract you. If they qualify, then they might be good to study with. That way, you'll have people to take breaks and eat your meals with. You'll also feel like you're not alone in your studying. Misery loves company!

- **Classmates:** When you are just beginning to study for exams, it's not really a good idea to study with your classmates. You need time to tackle the material on your own. Often, classmates will only serve to make you nervous for no good reason. They'll also take up a lot of your time by asking you questions before you've even had a chance to learn the material. It's better to work on the information by yourself first and call someone if you need help later.

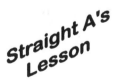 Studying with your friends isn't a bad idea as long as they're considerate. Studying with classmates, on the other hand, might not be as beneficial. They'll probably just create useless stress for you.

Get Out Of Your Home

We've talked about where to study and with whom. Here is my last piece of advice for this chapter: Get out of your apartment or home when you're studying for exams. Here's my reasoning:

- **Distractions:** Even if you pull out your phone and lock your door, there are still many more distractions at home than at a library.

- **Change of scenery:** If you're stuck in your house studying for long periods of time, you're going to get really bored looking at your four walls. Spending the day at a library and then returning home in the evening will create a pleasant change of scenery for you.

- **Get outside:** The fresh air on the way to the library, even if it's just walking from the parking lot to the front door, will help clear your mind.

- **Sleep:** If you're studying all day in your room, it will become a stressful environment for you and you might tense up when you're in it. As a result, you may find it difficult to fall asleep at night. A better idea is to leave your room for the day. Then, when you're finished studying, return home. You'll put your head down on your pillow and have no trouble getting to sleep.

- **Motivation:** Seeing other people studying around you at the library will motivate you.

- **Help is all around you:** If you run into any problems, you'll probably be able to find someone in the library to help you out.

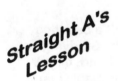

There are many reasons why you should get out of your apartment or house when you want to do serious studying.

The Night Before The Exam

- Finish your studying early and relax.
- Go to bed early.
- Make sure you have all the things you need for the exam such as identification, pencils/pens, water bottle, etc.
- Double-check the time and location of your exam.
- Set two alarms to ensure you wake up on time.

The Morning Of The Exam

- Review your notes.
- Make sure you know formulas, acronyms and lists.
- Eat a balanced breakfast.
- Go to the exam a little early.
- Double check you have everything you need.
- Go to the washroom before you go into the exam.
- Dress in layers so you won't boil if it's really hot in the exam room.

Exercise

Visualize Yourself Walking Into The Exam

I'll give you a little trick that my mother would suggest to me when I called her nervous about an upcoming exam:

1. Lie down on your bed in a comfortable position.
2. Picture yourself walking into the exam. Think about the clothes you're wearing, the bag you're carrying, even the look on your face. You want to make this picture very vivid in your mind.
3. Then, picture yourself actually walking into the room where you will be writing your exam.
4. You're now looking over the exam. You breathe a sigh of relief realizing that you know almost all the answers to the questions.
5. Your mind is focused as you sit writing the exam. You are confident you're going to ace it.
6. Finally, imagine yourself handing in the exam. You casually grin to yourself because you know how prepared you were. You leave the exam room and walk out. All went as well as you had planned.

Many people believe that if you visualize yourself doing something, and you make this visualization vivid enough so that it appears realistic to you, then you increase the chances that the visualization will turn into reality. It's known as a self-fulfilling prophecy and that's really what we're trying to do here. Picturing yourself walking confidently into an exam and acing it will help calm your nerves and give you the positive attitude you need on the day of your exam. Try this exercise out for yourself. It will only take a minute and it will help you get focused on succeeding in your exam.

Summary

After reading this chapter, you should feel all set for exam time. I've given you some tips on how to make life bearable, and even enjoyable, during exam time. We've also gone over the importance of keeping calm. If you're going to get stressed out during exam time, do it early and get it out of the way so you can get down to studying. By the night before your exam, you should have little left to do. Don't worry if you're stomach is filled with butterflies on the day of the exam. It could help you to perform your best.

Next we discussed the importance of getting into a routine. I suggested that you use the *ten o'clock rule* – finish studying by ten so you have time to relax before going to bed. You've got to have some fun on the weekends and include breaks when you study. Finally, we talked about where and with whom you should be studying, and the importance of getting out of your home. If you keep these things in mind, you should have no trouble surviving exam time.

CHAPTER 9

WRITE EFFECTIVE ESSAYS

Much more terrifying for me than writing exams, was writing a university paper. Sure, I had written several papers in high school, but this was a whole new ball game. In high school, classes were small and my teachers told me exactly what they wanted in my essays. In university, however, I was suddenly given topics to write about and very few instructions.

Writing papers in university was a new experience for me and it took a while before I become adept at it. Now, after four years of undergraduate studies, I feel I know all the ins and outs of writing effective papers. By my last year in university, I had created a step-by-step process for paper writing that never failed to get me the top marks I was aiming for. I am going to share that process with you very soon.

In this chapter, I'll present a complete explanation of how you should be writing your essays and papers. **First**, I'll go over the preliminary things to think about when you get a paper assigned. They include starting right away, making a timetable for yourself, and categorizing your essay according to its length and type, and the course it's for. **Next**, I'll give you a method of writing essays that includes choosing a topic, doing the research, and actually getting down to writing it. The **final** section is probably the most important. It's about the editing stage of paper writing and includes three important steps: Reorganizing your information, correcting your writing style, and getting a second editor. Once you have a handle on these things, you'll feel a lot more confident in your ability to write an excellent paper.

Preliminary Remarks

You've just been assigned an essay. It's due in a month. However, before you shove it aside and decide to pull an all-nighter right before it's due, let me try to convince you otherwise.

Start Right Away

You really don't need to be Hemingway in order to write a winning essay. What you do need, however, is time. Writing a good essay is very time consuming and with all of your other responsibilities at university, this can become a major problem.

The easiest way around this potential problem is to start your essay right away. That means that as soon as you get your essay assigned, you should start thinking about it. As long as you start far enough in advance, you'll have no problem budgeting your time. However, if you put your essay off, you just won't be able to dedicate the amount of time you'll need to write it well and your mark will suffer miserably as a result.

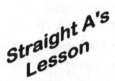

Start your essay as soon as you can. That way, you'll have enough time to devote to your paper without cutting too much into your other responsibilities.

Make A Timetable For Yourself

If you want to get a paper done on time, you need a plan of attack. Therefore, the first thing to do when assigned a paper is to make a timetable.

You want to be specific when making your timetable. That is, you want to indicate when you plan to complete each step in the essay writing process. This will provide you with checkpoints to judge whether you are on schedule as time passes, allowing you to adjust your working habits accordingly.

Here is a worksheet that you can use to assist you in making a schedule for writing your essay:

	Begin	Finish
1. Choose topic	_____	_____
2. Research	_____	_____
3. Read research	_____	_____
4. Take notes	_____	_____
5. Organize research	_____	_____
6. Make outline for essay	_____	_____
7. Draft 1 of essay	_____	_____
8. Draft 2 of essay	_____	_____
9. Draft ___ of essay	_____	_____
10. Edit essay	_____	_____
11. Hand in Essay	_____	

An essay is usually assigned at least four to six weeks in advance of its due date if it requires significant research. When you make up your schedule, you should always plan to finish your essay, with all of the editing completed, at least a week early. That way, you'll give yourself enough time to add any last minute ideas, to make corrections, or to talk to your professor about any concerns you're having.

Once your timetable is established, you'll have a good idea of *what* you should be doing and *when* you should be doing it. It's not imperative that you stick to your schedule religiously, but it is important you have a guideline to help you meet your deadlines and get a sense of your progress.

Your essay timetable is not written in stone. As you move along, you'll likely need to make some adjustments.

Straight A's Lesson

You must create a schedule for writing your essay that includes all the various steps in the process. This will give you deadlines to adhere to and help you to keep on track. It will also ensure that you've left yourself enough time to go through the required essay writing steps.

Categorize The Essay

Thus far, I have used the term essay very broadly. The truth is essays can vary significantly in terms of length and style. While the basic method that I discuss in the next section applies to all essays, there are some things you should know about each specific kind of essay.

When you are assigned an essay, you should try to categorize it as a preliminary step. This will help you to determine how much time and effort will be required to write an 'A' paper. You should categorize the essay according to its length, the type of essay, and the course the essay is for.

Length of essay: There are different things you should think about when preparing to write your essay that depend on how long the essay is required to be.

- **1-2 Page Essay** (250-500 words):
- Little or no research needed.
- Stick to the point.
- Edit away any extraneous information.
- Every word counts so be careful and choose words appropriately.
- Very short introduction and conclusion.
- You'll spend more time editing these essays than actually writing them.

- **5-10 Pages**
- Research needed.
- More detail and specifics than in a 1-2 page essay.
- Stick to a thesis / main point throughout essay.
- Longer introduction and conclusion.
- Use a few headings within your paper to help organize it. Headings are titles within essays that indicate the general area that will be discussed in the next few paragraphs.

- **10-30 Pages**
- Time-consuming but not difficult.
- Much research needed.
- Organization within the paper is key! Use a lot of headings and sub-headings. (Sub-headings are headings that categorize information under headings.)

- You can argue a thesis point and then sub-points as well throughout your essay.
- Introduction should be thorough, giving the reader a road map to the essay. Conclusion should shed light on the importance of the topic in a larger perspective.

Type of essay: The two main types of essays that you will come across at university I refer to as thesis and expository.

- In a thesis-based essay, you are trying to prove a point or an argument. This is a very directed essay in that the information you provide should somehow prove or disprove the thesis presented.

- In an expository essay, you want to concentrate on explaining a concept, idea, or event rather than on making an argument about a certain topic. For example, you might be presenting an account of the events that occurred during a World War without making an argument for or against them.

- In university or college, you'll probably deal with thesis-based essays most often. These are a little more difficult than expository essays. First, you must do research on a topic. Then, you must try to prove or disprove an argument relating to that topic. I have found that these essays take a lot more effort and time than expository essays. However, they can be a lot more personally rewarding than expository essays since they challenge you to think more deeply and creatively about a particular topic.

Type of course: You might want to structure your essay according to the type of course it is for. Here are some points to think about:

- **English essays:** Some people get carried away writing English essays by trying to make them creative, eloquent, and full of literary devices. I suggest that when writing English essays, you should begin by focusing primarily on the content of the paper. Later, you can work on sprucing it up and making it more poetic.

- **Philosophy essays:** If you remember the three C's to writing philosophy papers you'll have no problem. Make sure your paper is clear, concise, and concrete.

- *Clear*: Go through each line in your essay to make sure that what you're trying to get across is clear to the reader. You want to avoid any ambiguity.

- *Concise*: Philosophers spent their lives writing lengthy explanations for all their ideas. You don't have to follow their lead. Professors want to see that you can explain something efficiently, using as few words as possible. Spend time editing your papers to avoid useless rambling.

- *Concrete*: A lot of philosophical concepts are complex. The challenge in writing a philosophy paper is to explain these concepts as clearly and simply as possible.

- **Mathematical/Scientific Essays:** In these essays you'll probably be required to include scientific information or mathematical formulas. You'll need to get a computer program (if your computer doesn't come with one) that is capable of writing formulas and scientific expressions. You want to pay careful attention to precision in these essays, ensuring that all the information and calculations are accurate.

- **Social Science Essays:** Here's a tip that's really helped me in my social science classes: 'More is better'. But I'm not necessarily talking about length here. The more involved you get in your paper, the more research you do, and the more you read over and edit your paper, the more likely it will be highly appraised by your professor. You don't need to be brilliant to write an excellent social science essay. However, you have to be willing to immerse yourself in the topic and spend some quality time researching it. At the same time, you still have to find that optimal time to quit your research so you can begin writing the actual essay. Your timetable will come in handy as far as sticking to your deadlines.

Straight A's Lesson

When you're assigned an essay, as a preliminary step, you should categorize it according to its length, the type of essay it is, and the type of course the essay is for. This will give you some sense of how much time and effort your essay will require.

That concludes my introductory remarks about essays. By now you should have some idea what you have to do when you're assigned an essay. It's time now to move on and learn about my personal method to writing essays.

Method To Essay Writing

Like everything else in university, employing a method will make essay writing much more simple and make getting a top mark a lot more likely. There are three main steps involved in writing an essay that I'll discuss. They are, choosing your topic, doing the research, and writing the paper. Within each step, there are certain things you need to do. I've outlined them in the sections that follow.

Topic Choice

Scenario: You're assigned an essay and by next week you're supposed to choose your topic and hand it in to your professor. For several days though, you do nothing. Then, on the eve of your deadline, you briefly consider what topic to choose for your essay. You thoughtlessly jot down a topic and hand it over to your professor the next day.

This is a common scenario. I've approached things this way myself many times. However, it's really not a good idea. The problem is that you'll likely end up being stuck writing about something you didn't choose with much thought. It's possible that you won't be able to grasp your topic because it's beyond your comprehension. Worse yet, you may find that most of the research material on your topic is only available in a foreign language. When you finally discover what you're up against, you'll be sorry you didn't take the time to choose a topic more carefully.

It's much better to choose a topic that you find interesting and that you think you'll be able to do a good job on. Following is the method I suggest you use when choosing your topic:

- **Talk to your professor**: Once you have some ideas about what kind of topic you'd like to do, talk to your professor to find out which of your ideas will be interesting and easy to research. Pick out three that your professor approves of and then go to step 2.

- **Pre-topic research**: Do some quick research on your prospective topics. Decide which topic interests you the most (your topic really has to stimulate you for you to write an effective paper). By the end of this step, you should have a general topic for your paper.

- **Narrow the topic**: Once you have chosen your general topic, try to narrow it down by researching the topic a little more and talking, once again, to your professor. By narrowing the topic down, you'll ensure that your essay is tightly knit and sharply focused. Here's a tip that may help you when you're narrowing your topic: Come up with an interesting question about your general topic – something that whets your curiosity – and then go ahead and answer it. In a nutshell, that's your paper!

At the end of these three easy steps, you should have a feasible topic for your essay. Now it's time to get to the meat of the essay writing method – the research.

Straight A's Lesson

When choosing your topic for a paper, talk to your professor, do some preliminary research, and narrow down your topic choice. Be sure to complete these three steps quickly so you can begin to work on the actual essay as soon as possible.

Researching Your Topic

Learning The Library: When you begin university or college, I strongly suggest that you find the time to learn your way around the library. At the beginning of the year, there are usually library information sessions. While others may view anyone who attends these as a 'loser', you'll feel like a winner down the road when it comes time to do research for your papers.

If you attend one of these sessions, by the time you have to begin researching a paper, you should already have a fairly good sense of how to use the computers, conduct searches, and locate books and articles. If you're unable to retain all the knowledge you learn in the library information session, there are always librarians around who are just waiting to help people like you who feel lost. Don't hesitate to ask for help whenever you need it.

Straight A's Lesson

Learn your way around your school's library either by attending information sessions at the beginning of the school year or by asking librarians for assistance when you need it. You should become adept at using the various computers and search engines as they will save you time when you have to do research.

Start Right Away

Researching can be a pain! You may find that it takes you a while before you come close to finding the information you're looking for. You may also find that the library at your university doesn't have the proper information and you'll need to go to a different one in the area.

Whatever the reason, your research can take a lot more of your time than you had anticipated. Therefore, as soon as you've chosen your topic, get yourself to the library. Begin your research as soon as possible because you never know what kind of problems you might encounter.

Straight A's Lesson

Start your research as soon as you've chosen your topic. That way, even if you run into problems, you'll still have enough time to do all the research you need to get that 'A'.

The Seven Steps To Researching

There is a seven-step process that you should follow when doing your research. You can modify these steps based on the type of essay you're writing.

1. **Get references from your professor:** After you choose your topic, the first thing you should do is go to your professor to ask where you should start your research. Your professor will likely suggest a few articles or books for you to begin with. You should take the time to read through these sources and familiarize yourself with the topic and the lingo.

2. **Expand your research:** You should now have a handle on the topic. It's time to expand your research. You can do this in two easy steps.

    - Use the bibliographies of the sources you already have to find more information pertinent to your topic.
    - Do a search on the library computer system.

    As you gather information, skim it over to find what's useful for you. Here are some things to look for:

    - **Date:** Usually the more recent the material is, the better it will be for your paper.
    - **Author:** Check out who wrote the book or article. Look into the author's qualifications to see whether he or she has been recognized by others who are respected in the field.
    - **Argumentative:** You will get a different perspective on the topic based on whether the sources are argumentative (trying to prove a point), biased, or more objective (i.e. most textbooks). You want to get a variety of perspectives when writing a paper.
    - **Abstract:** Most articles will contain an abstract that summarizes the information presented. Reading the abstract is a quick way to determine whether the article can be useful to you.

3. **Read sources:** By now, you should have gathered a lot of articles and books for your essay. It's time to sit back and start reading. If you're reading from photocopies, it's a good idea to highlight important points as you read. If you're reading books however, use labeled Post-it™ notes

to mark where important information is located. When reading
through your sources, keep these things in mind:

- Think about a thesis: You already have a narrow topic that you're
  researching, but now you want to determine a thesis: one sentence
  that concisely sums up what you're trying to prove in your paper.
  While you're reading through your sources, play around with a
  possible thesis in the back of your mind. As you get ideas, jot them
  down so you don't forget them.

- Familiarize yourself: You'll want to acquire a solid understanding of
  your topic. That's why it's important to take the time to read your
  sources carefully. Even if you still don't understand everything
  word for word, just getting a sense of what it's all about will be
  helpful. Learning the 'lingo' surrounding a certain topic is also
  important if you plan on writing an impressive paper.

- Categorize the information: Get a sense of what sources give what
  kind of information. Some sources will give you background
  information, some will present an argument, and others will present
  statistical proof. Making note of which sources present which kind
  of information on your topic will be helpful when you begin to take
  notes from your sources.

4. **Choose a thesis:** By now, you've done enough reading to give you some
   idea of what you'll be trying to prove or disprove in your paper. Talk to
   your professor (or teaching assistant/fellow) about your idea and get
   their input. They'll probably help you refine it and together you'll
   come up with a clear thesis and the best wording of it. This is a very
   good thing to do! Getting your professor or teaching assistant/fellow to
   agree on your thesis will make getting the grade you want much more
   likely.

5. **Take notes:** You've now read a lot of source material and you feel like
   you have a solid grasp on the information presented. It's time to take
   out your notebook and pen and start taking notes. This is a very
   important step that many students overlook. Here are some things to
   consider:

- Start with what's most important: Since you've already read your source material, you have an idea of what is most pertinent to your topic. Begin to take notes from those sources and work your way down to the material that's least important.

- Divide and conquer: You'll likely feel as if there is so much information in front of you that there's no way you can get through it all. I suggest that when you start to take notes, you put away all of your sources except for the book or article you are using. Concentrate only on what's in front of you so that you don't get overwhelmed.

- Organize your notes: When taking notes, you want to start categorizing the information contained therein. Do this by taking notes under clear headings. When it's time to actually write your paper, you'll be able to quickly find the information you're looking for.

- Be thorough: If you're writing a fairly long essay, you'll want to be quite thorough in your research. Go through the sources slowly enough so that you catch what's important. Understand what you are reading and write things accurately into your notes. If you want more information on a certain portion of your source material, look at the article's bibliography and search out the sources referred to. This will make for a comprehensive paper.

- Don't copy word for word: A major point of note taking is that it gives you the chance to put things into your own words. This will help you grasp what you're reading and ensure that your paper won't sound too similar to your sources.

- Keep a good record of sources used: Whenever you take notes from a source, even if you're not using exact quotes, clearly indicate which books or articles you are using and the page from which the information was taken. This will make footnoting your essay a simple thing to do.

6. **Read over and organize your notes**: Now that you have all of the notes from your sources, it's time to get organized. First, review your notes by skimming through them. Then, put your notes into some sort of order

by gathering all the related information together. If you can't physically rearrange your notes, just take a red marker and indicate at the top of each page what type of information is there.

7. **Make an outline**: Once you've organized your information, you'll have some idea of the specific areas that you'll discuss in your paper. Start to create an outline by arranging these different areas of discussion into a logical order. You'll begin your paper with an introduction and you'll end it with a conclusion. What appears in between depends on the information you've gathered. When creating your outline, consider the following:

    *   Background information: If you're writing a fairly long essay, make sure that you present background information on your topic. This background information should follow right after your introduction. You want to be sure that even a completely uninformed reader would be able to follow along, understanding your essay. That's why it's important to lay out a foundation for the topic. Remember: You've researched this topic for over a month, the person reading it, however, has not.

    *   Logical presentation: Present the information in your paper in a logical way. For example, if you are discussing historical events, use a chronological format. Or, if your essay is on a certain industry, explain the industry's structure before delving into problems that the industry encounters. Whatever your order of presenting information is, make sure one topic develops logically from the topic preceding it.

    *   All points should go back to the thesis: If you are trying to prove a thesis, make sure that most of the information you're planning to discuss relates clearly to the thesis.

Straight A's Lesson

There are seven easy steps to doing good research. They are: getting sources from your professor, expanding your research, reading your sources, choosing your thesis, taking notes, organizing your notes, and making an outline. Following these steps will get you well prepared for writing the actual essay.

Once you've finished creating an outline for your paper, you've completed the seven easy steps to researching. You're now ready to put your pen to paper (or fingers to keyboard if you're using a computer) to begin writing your essay.

Writing Your Paper

The actual writing of your paper can seem like the most difficult part of the essay writing process. Sitting in front of a large, blank, computer screen can be very intimidating. Even today, I still feel nervous when I start to write a paper, regardless of its length or difficulty level. However, writing your paper can be simple if you learn the techniques I've discovered and practiced over the years.

a) Just Write

The best way to avoid writer's block is simply to stop thinking and start writing. Your notes are in front of you, your outline is staring you in the face, and your computer screen is wired up. It's time to write!

Write your first draft as quickly as possible and don't worry about perfecting it at this stage. Spelling mistakes, grammatical errors, and problems with explanations can all be fixed later. You just want to have a completed first draft as quickly as possible. That way, a lot of the stress of getting something down on paper is out of the way and, no matter what, you'll at least have something that *could* be handed in. Once you've written this first draft, you can gradually work on transforming it from one that's not so great into one that you'll be proud of.

Straight A's Lesson

Write a quick first draft. Then, you'll be less stressed about writing your paper and you'll be able to concentrate on improving it.

b) Writing Your First Draft

You want to get your first draft written right away and there's a way that you should go about doing it. First, you have to divide up your whole paper into three smaller sections – the introduction, the body, and the conclusion – so you can work on it one piece at a time.

Introduction

Here are the basics to writing an introduction:

- General introductory remarks: Begin your essay with interesting comments that relate broadly to your topic.

- Thesis statement: This is a statement of intent, what you're trying to prove in your essay. Lead into your thesis statement from your general introductory remarks.

- Outline of paper: In your introduction, you want to inform the reader what you will be discussing in your paper and the order in which you will be discussing it.

As long as you include these three things in your introduction, it should be adequate. On the first draft, don't worry too much about getting it perfect. Just write something down for now and come back to it later.

The Body

Since you've already written the outline of your paper (step 7 in **Steps to Researching**), you'll already have logically divided the body of your essay into the sections that you will be discussing. Now it's easy – just pick a section and write it.

How do you write a section of your essay? Well, to begin with, write down the heading at the top of your screen or paper and then gather the notes you've written that relate to that section. Review them briefly and then pick an area to discuss and write down information as it comes to you.

In my approach to writing papers, first and foremost, is to just get it finished. Then, all you're left with is the task of improving it. The following are some tips to remember when writing each section in the body of your essay:

- *Write one section at a time*: As long as you divide the information into sections, it will be much easier for you to write. Writing a long paper doesn't seem as difficult or stressful when you tackle it bit by bit.

- *Use headings*: When you're writing the body of your paper, use headings that clearly label the information you're presenting. This will keep your paper both organized and focused. Your job will seem like a breeze.

- *Footnote*: Don't forget to include footnotes in your first draft. You want to get into the habit of footnoting every piece of information you take from a source. By doing it right away, you won't have to waste your time later on with this tedious technicality. However, your footnotes don't have to be perfect in your first draft. Just get down the information you want and worry about the precision of them later.

- *Use your own words*: Take a step back from your notes and try to explain things as much as you can in your own words. It's obvious to the professor reading your paper whether you know what you're talking about or whether you've just reworded and rearranged information straight out of a book.

Conclusion

In the introduction of your paper, tell the reader what it is you're planning to discuss and in the body be sure to stick to this idea. Then, in the conclusion reiterate everything you've discussed to make it perfectly clear for the reader. Clarity is the most basic element of a well-written paper.

In the conclusion, first restate the thesis statement using different wording than you used in the introduction. Next, briefly review the information that you presented in the essay. Finally, put your essay topic into a much larger framework, showing how it relates to a much bigger picture. All of these elements make for a satisfying conclusion. (Side note: Try to avoid opening your conclusion with the words "In conclusion..." Many professors find it 'elementary'.)

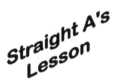

When writing your first draft, start with the introduction, continue to the body of the essay, and finish with the conclusion. When composing the body, write one section of your outline at a time.

See Your Professor

After you have your first draft written, you should see your professor or teaching assistant/fellow to discuss it. Bring a copy of your first draft when you go. This visit will accomplish three important things:

- It will show them that you're working hard on the essay. You already have a rough draft completed well ahead of your assignment deadline.

- It will give you an opportunity to listen to any suggestions your teacher may have for improving your essay (i.e. organization, content, or thesis improvements).

- It will give you some idea of how much work your paper still needs before completion. You'll find out if you still need to do more research or if you can go right to the editing phase. Whatever the case, because you've completed the rough draft so quickly, you'll have plenty of time to do what needs to be done to make improvements.

Straight A's Lesson

Take your first draft to your teacher to look over. Your teacher may give you helpful advice as to what you should be doing next.

Hurray! You have completed a rough draft of your essay. Suddenly, your essay doesn't seem so difficult and your nervousness subsides. However, don't think you're home free just yet. You still have a big job ahead of you that will ultimately determine the grade you receive on your paper. It's time to edit. Let's begin...

Editing Your Paper

It's the editing of your paper that will either make or break your chances for a decent grade. Be sure to leave yourself enough time to do a solid editing job.

Reorganizing Your Essay

The first thing to worry about in the editing stage of your essay writing process is getting all the information presented in a logical and coherent manner. Since I suggested that you write your first draft quickly, you likely didn't present things in the best way you could have. That's okay. You still have a lot of time to rearrange things during the editing phase of your paper.

I can't imagine what essay writing was like in the days before computers. My favorite tool to use on the computer is the 'cut and paste' function, which allows you to easily reorganize your material as much as you need to. You want everything to fit just perfectly. Play around with how to paste all your material together for maximum coherence. You'll find that if you experiment a little, you'll get a much more concise and organized essay.

Now you should have the information laid out just the way you want it. However, during the reorganizing stage, you might also want to:

- **Add information or remove large chunks**: You should be able to tell by now what information is useful to your paper and what material serves merely to confuse the reader. You'll likely also see where you need more information, either to support a point or provide a more detailed explanation of something. If you still need to do a little more research, it's not a problem. Quite often, it's those last few efforts you make that really ensure your paper stands out from the rest of the pile.

- **Make sure one paragraph flows logically to the next**: A good essay flows well; each paragraph seems to fall perfectly into the appropriate place. Making this happen is easy! The trick to this is that you want to connect each paragraph to the previous one. You can do this in the first line of each paragraph by using hook words such as 'in addition to', 'as well', 'conversely', 'on the other hand', 'first of all', 'second of all', etc. Another way to ensure your paper flows is to use a pronoun in the first sentence of a new paragraph that refers to the previous paragraph. For example, you might start a new paragraph by writing, 'Following **this** line of reasoning... '.

- **Make sure sections in your essay flow logically into each other**: Sections refer to chunks of information presented under a heading. You can make one section flow nicely into the next by using a lead-in line. In other words, make the last sentence of one section a preview for the section that follows. This prepares the reader for what it is you're about to discuss (see the last sentence of Chapter Six for an example of a lead-in line). Another way to seamlessly join each section is by using a connecting paragraph at the beginning of a new section that gradually moves the reader from one topic into the next.

Improving Your Writing Style

By now, you should have the information in your paper completely organized. It's finally time to put on the finishing touches. An essay is not the same as an assignment or an exam where you're usually not graded on diction, style, or spelling. However, all of these things count in an essay, so take time to improve your writing style.

To improve the writing style in your paper, you'll want to concentrate on the following:

- **Spelling:** The 'spell check' feature on your computer should be able to catch most of your spelling errors. However, consider that there might be many words in your paper that are spelled properly but used incorrectly. For example, you might write 'principle' when you mean to write 'principal'. These words will not appear as being wrong on your 'spell check' because they are spelled correctly. But obviously, they mean very different things. You want to pay careful attention to ensure that you not only spell words correctly but also that you use them properly.

- **Grammar:** The 'grammar check' feature on your computer can be helpful, but you really do need to read your paper carefully in order to solve all of your grammatical problems. If you're not confident in your own ability to catch your dangling participles, misplaced modifiers, and faulty parallel structures, you might want to check out the web sites that I list under "Essay Writing Websites" in the back of this book. Many of them give quick tutorials on English grammar. As well, you'll want to have someone else correct your paper. (I talk about the importance of a second editor in the next section.)

- **Diction:** You certainly don't need to use words that are thirty letters long, but you do need to use words appropriately. Choose words carefully so that they help to convey the point you're trying to make. Obviously, the larger the vocabulary you have, the easier it will be to do this. Reading books and looking up the words that you don't understand can help improve your vocabulary dramatically. But, make sure that whenever you use a word that you're not completely familiar with, you look it up in the dictionary to ensure that it actually means what you think. It's quite evident to a professor reading your paper if you are relying on your computer's thesaurus function.

- **Sentence Variation:** If every sentence in your essay contains a subject, followed by a verb, followed by an object, your essay will end up being quite boring to read. Try sprucing up your sentence structure by rearranging the word order in some sentences. You can begin to do this by moving some prepositions to the beginning of your sentences. For example, instead of writing, "Sally went to the park in the middle of the day," you could write, "In the middle of the day, Sally went to the park." Keep in mind that varying your sentence structure makes for a more enjoyable read.

- **Readability:** Read a paper out loud to make sure that it flows. If it doesn't read well, add in a syllable or word here or there.

- **Punctuation:** Make sure you are using periods, commas, semi-colons, and question marks properly so that your paper reads sensibly.

These are some basic things to remember when you're trying to improve your writing style. The way in which you write your essay can be almost as important as the information you write about. If your professor is constantly finding spelling and grammatical mistakes, he or she might underestimate the extent of the research you've done and the quality of the information that you've presented. You don't want this to happen, especially since most spelling and grammatical errors are easy to fix. Simply read over your paper a couple of times carefully and look for them.

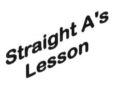

The way in which you write your essay can be almost as important as the information you write about. Pay attention to your grammar.

Getting A Second Editor

You've probably read over your paper so many times that you can no longer pick up on the obvious mistakes that are often right under your nose. It's possible to be too familiar with your paper and, as a result, you may not be able to recognize a missing word or an improper punctuation mark. That's why a second editor is helpful.

As a general rule, you should never hand in a paper that has not been edited by someone other than yourself. It's essential that you find someone who is proficient in the English language (or whatever language your paper is written in). However, your editor need not be overly familiar with your topic. I've listed some suggestions of people who you could ask to be your second editor:

- Family members
- Friends
- Websites – There are some sites where you can have your papers edited for a fee. I list a few under "Essay Writing" at the back of the book.

- Tutor – It is possible to hire someone at your school to help you edit your papers.
- English Department – Most schools set up a free editing service in their English department. Find out if your school has one and use it.

Plagiarizing

The surest way to ruin your university career is by plagiarizing. Copying an idea, a sentence, or even just a phrase from a source without properly citing it is illegal. It can easily get you kicked out of university. Avoid it at all costs!

That's not to say you can't make use of other people's ideas, words, and concepts. In fact, you should include 'borrowed' ideas as long as you reference them accordingly. Use footnotes or endnotes wherever you've taken someone else's idea.

My rule of thumb is that it's better to 'over footnote' than 'under footnote'. If you're unsure whether or not you should reference something or someone, do it regardless.

Footnotes

Footnotes can seem terribly complicated if you haven't had much experience writing papers. However, if you have specific directions on how to properly cite your sources, it becomes a cinch. At the back of this book, I list various websites that show you how to set up your footnotes according to the MLA (Modern Language Association) style. If your professors don't give you a specific format that they'd like you to employ, use the websites that I've listed. These sites have the most recent information on how to footnote both traditional sources as well as Internet/electronic sources.

Remember: Whatever method of footnotes you choose to use, consistency is the key. As long as you follow a consistent system of citing your sources, your professor will probably accept it.

Finishing Touches

Once your essay has been edited to death, it's time to put it all together into a presentable finished product. Here are some things to remember:

- **Title page**: You want to make sure you have all of the required information on your title page such as the title of your paper, your name, your professor's name, the date, and the course number.

- **Number your pages**: All professors want you to number your pages just in case the pages get shuffled around.

- **Binding**: Whenever I hand in a fairly lengthy paper, I always have it bound. Binding makes a paper look professional and shows the professor that you're putting in that extra bit of effort.

- **Graphs and tables**: If your paper calls for graphs and tables, you can either include them within the body of the paper or refer to them in the appendices. Make sure you label them appropriately so that they are easy to locate within your paper.

- **Footnotes and endnotes**: You need to take extra care to properly cite all of your sources.

Summary Of Steps To Writing The Perfect Paper

Choose Your Topic
- Talk to your professor
- Pre-topic research
- Narrow down your topic

Do Your Research
- Start with sources that your professor recommends
- Expand your research
- Read through your sources
- Articulate a thesis for your paper
- Take notes on your sources
- Organize your notes
- Create the outline for your essay

Write Your Paper
- Write your first draft quickly
- See your professor with your first draft

Edit Your Paper
- Reorganize the information in your essay
- Improve your writing style
- Get a second editor

Commonly Asked Questions

Question: When I have an essay to write for a class, should I look over the essays of others who have previously taken the same class?

Answer: You've really got to be careful when it comes to essay writing. The worst thing you can do is copy an essay off of a friend. First of all, it's illegal and you'll likely get caught. A lot of professors photocopy old essays and keep them on record. Besides, writing essays is one of the most important skills you'll learn in university. It's a skill that will come in handy over and over again throughout your education and career.

Summary

There you have it! It's all you've ever wanted to know about writing the perfect essay. I began by giving you some preliminary advice: Start your essay as soon as it's assigned, make a timetable for yourself, and categorize the essay. Then I gave you my complete and comprehensive method to essay writing that includes choosing a topic, conducting the research, and writing the paper. Finally, I focused on the importance of the editing stage in the essay writing process. You really want to make sure that you've reorganized the information as best as possible, have corrected the writing style, and have used a second editor to make further corrections. As long as you follow the techniques I've presented, you'll have no problem writing a first class essay.

CHAPTER 10

GET A LIFE OUTSIDE OF SCHOOL

Imagine your daily life at school. You wake up every morning, go to class, come home and open your books to study, and then go to sleep. You repeat this same routine day after day. Even though we understand that you need to put in your fair share of studying to get the grades you're after, you'll be very disappointed at the end of your school years if that's the *only* thing that you've done. The point here is that you should make sure that you have a life outside of school.

University/college is a good time to meet people from all over the world. It's a chance to experience new things and to learn about yourself in a whole new way. In this chapter, I'll emphasize the value of making the most of your school experience. **First**, I'll stress the importance of being a well-rounded person. This includes making friends, getting involved in extracurricular and volunteer activities, and finding great summer jobs. **Second**, I'll tell you how important it is to take care of yourself at school by eating right, exercising, and getting enough sleep. **Finally**, I'll tell you about the importance of putting everything in perspective. This involves realizing that there are many second chances in school, creating outlets for stress relief, and deciding to compete only with yourself. Making the most of your whole school experience will leave you with fond memories of these exciting years.

Be Well-Rounded

Sitting in your room and studying day and night will help you with your grades, but it won't help you much when you apply to graduate programs or look for jobs. While good grades can help open doors to opportunities, employers and school administrators also want to know you communicate well with others, have interests outside of school, and have a history of positive employment experiences. These are important things to consider during your years in school. Don't overlook them!

Make Friends

When you go to school, you can expect to learn a ton of important information from your professors, from the books you read, and from the enormous library on campus. What you might not expect is that some of the most important insights you'll gain will come from the people you pass in the hallways or sit next to in the cafeteria. That's right, the people you meet in school can be your most inspiring sources of knowledge. However, it's not likely you'll meet them sitting locked up in your room.

If you come to school with an open mind, eager to cross paths with interesting people, then this will just evolve naturally. However, if you're having trouble meeting the type of people you want, then you might have to make a conscious effort to do so. Start by getting involved with different organizations or clubs.

The point here is that you've got to get out there and make a life for yourself. Meeting people is an important part of that life, and university is full of opportunities.

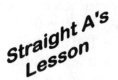

Some of the most important things you'll learn in school will come from the people you'll meet. Be friendly and try to develop a wide range of relationships.

Get Involved In Extracurricular And Volunteer Activities

There are so many reasons why you should get involved in extracurricular and volunteer activities. Here are just a few:

- You'll meet a lot of people.
- You'll build up your self-confidence and acquire a sense of self worth by seeing that you're a contributor to important causes.
- You'll have a resume that graduate program administrators and job interviewers will notice.
- It will give you a needed break from your schoolwork.

You probably have you own reasons for wanting to get involved in school or in your community. Even if you're not quite convinced of the positive benefits of doing so, trust me and try it out.

My own experience of volunteering in the community around my university introduced me to many interesting people that I wouldn't have met otherwise. It also helped me gain leadership skills, taught me about responsibility, and brought me awards and scholarships that helped pay for my university education. Simply put, my university experience would not have been as rewarding without volunteering.

Straight A's Lesson

Get involved in university by joining clubs, volunteering, or finding your own activities. It will introduce you to interesting people, develop your personality, and help you in the future when you're looking for jobs and applying to graduate programs.

Get Great Summer Jobs

In between your years in school, there'll be a few months to do as you wish. Still, even if you're one of the rare few who don't need the money from a summer job, I suggest strongly that you get one regardless. The material you learn in school is of crucial value. However, I have yet to see any classes in school preparing their students for life in the working world. Summer jobs will offer you this knowledge. When you consider that summer jobs are only temporary, they never feel too oppressive. Before you know it, summer will be over and it will be time for you to head back to school. You may even be glad for it!

If you're still not convinced about the importance of getting a summer job, here are some other good reasons to show how beneficial they can be:

- Build up an impressive resume you'll use when applying for jobs or to graduate programs.
- Acquire practical skills.
- Network.
- Make money.

- Learn about communication and time management.
- Get used to the long hours of working.

There are obviously a lot of benefits from getting a summer job. However, actually getting these jobs might not be that easy, especially if you're still fairly young and do not have a lot of previous work experience. That's why it's important to think seriously about these things early on in your education.

If you can't find a summer job, consider volunteering or interning. If you do a good job there, you may actually be hired the following year. In any case, it will ensure you have a better resume to send out when applying for jobs.

Straight A's Lesson

Try to get summer jobs. They'll build up your resume and help you make important connections. If you can't get a job, try volunteering during the summer to build up your resume. Then, try applying again the following year.

Take Care Of Yourself While You're In School

You want to make the most of your university experience. However, that's pretty difficult to do if you're undernourished, inactive, or exhausted. There is just so much to do when you arrive at university and it all might feel overwhelming. It'll help if you make sure to take care of yourself. In this section I'll give you some pointers on things you should be doing to take care of yourself while in school.

Eat Right

A healthy body goes hand in hand with a healthy mind – one that works at maximum capacity. Don't overlook the importance of being properly nourished while in school. Here are some things to consider:

- **Don't overdose on junk food:** Junk food has a high sugar content that will give you an immediate burst of energy. However, because this boost of energy will subside quickly (the 'sugar slump'), you'll be left feeling very tired. It's difficult to concentrate when you're tired, especially where school is concerned.

- **Eat a lot of fresh fruits and vegetables:** They're full of vitamins and nutrients that will keep you healthy during your tiring school days.

- **Eat three meals a day:** Skipping meals will leave you tired, withdrawn and unable to concentrate properly.

- **Don't drink too much coffee:** Drinking too much coffee can cause morning headaches and this isn't a good thing, especially if you have to rush off to eight o'clock classes. Limit your coffee consumption to no more than two or three cups a day.

- **Take a multivitamin:** If you find that it's difficult to maintain a balanced diet, try taking a multivitamin that is high in B Vitamins (stress tends to deplete B vitamins in your body). This will ensure that you're still getting most of the nutrients you need even when you're on the go.

- **Always eat your breakfast:** It's tempting to skip your first meal so that you can get that extra ten minutes of sleep. But, eating a nutritious breakfast will give you a lot more energy than that extra ten minutes of sleep will. Having a solid breakfast will start your school days off right.

Straight A's Lesson

In order to enjoy your time in school and be able to concentrate on your studies, avoid illness by sticking to a balanced diet of three healthy meals a day.

Exercise

Rather than tiring you out, exercising can be invigorating. Don't eliminate exercise from your busy schedule since there are just too many benefits you can reap from it. Here are some benefits that you might not have considered:

- It's reenergizing.
- It can help you relieve stress.
- Great place to meet people (especially if you join intramural sports teams).
- Stay in shape.
- Relieves cramping and aching from sitting at your desk or computer.
- Helps to develop discipline.

Taking time out to exercise can relieve your stress and give you an energy boost. As a result, you'll find yourself much more able to concentrate and have a greater desire to work. I suggest exercising three times a week. It's a reasonable schedule that will be easy to stick to.

Straight A's Lesson

Try to exercise about three times a week. It will give you energy, relieve your stress, and it's a great way to meet people.

Sleep

An easy way to make time for everything you want to do in school is to decide to eliminate some of your sleep. You may think that if you sleep four hours instead of the eight you need, you'll be able to fit everything into your day just perfectly. Unfortunately, if you keep this up, you'll probably come crashing down by the middle of the semester, if not much sooner.

Keeping up a schedule that doesn't give you enough time to sleep is a great way to ruin your years in school. Not only will you be without the energy needed to concentrate, but you may also be unpleasant to be around. Whatever you do, consider sleep a priority in your life. To be able to function properly, you've got to get a good night's rest.

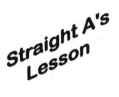

Make sure you take time in your busy schedule to get enough sleep on a daily basis.

Put Things In Perspective

It's easy to get caught up in the craziness that goes along with being a university or college student. At some point though, you've got to get your head together and put things in perspective. Here are some tips for doing just that.

There Are Many Second Chances

A very important thing to consider while you're in school is that there are a lot of second chances. Messing up one thing or another can happen to anyone. The important thing to remember in these instances is not to give up. Don't think, "I failed my midterm. There's no use now in trying to do well on the final!" That's a loser's attitude and will only hurt you in the long run.

If you keep in mind that there are a lot of second chances in school, you'll be less likely to let little mishaps discourage you. It's okay to screw up! It happens to the best of us. What isn't okay is to give up and not try anymore. Instead, realize that you have other chances to prove yourself and make the most of these opportunities.

Here are some things to illustrate what I mean by second chances in school:

- Let's say you bomb a midterm in a course, but then significantly improve on the final exam. It's possible that your professor will put more weight on your final exam than they were planning to when calculating your final grade. Talk to your professor about this possibility and explain why you had so much trouble on the midterm. Professors are human beings and can be understanding as long as you approach them diplomatically and sincerely.

- If you really fouled up on something in a particular course and are worried about your final grade, you can ask professors for an extra assignment or paper. If you appeal logically and persistently, they might consider it. Even if they don't concede, they will certainly take note that you really care about your final grade in the course. Who knows, they may even bump you up a percent or two.

- You take so many courses in school that even if you falter in a few of them, your overall grade point average may not be too damaged.

- If you totally mess up in your first year but from then on show a remarkable improvement, employers or graduate program administrators will take your improvement into consideration when looking at your transcript.

As you can see, there are a lot of second chances to be had in school. The important thing is that you recognize that these second chances exist, and go after them. If you get a result you're not especially happy with, just remember that the worst thing you can possibly do is throw in the towel.

Straight A's Lesson

There are a lot of second chances in school. Don't worry if you screw up. Through perseverance you should have no problem succeeding the next time.

Have Outlets To Relieve Your Stress

I am proud to say that I was able to succeed at university and, at least after my first year, maintain a certain level of calmness. My ability to do that relates to the outlets for stress reduction I was able to establish for myself. I made sure I had enough things in my life that were enjoyable to create a balance for my serious work schedule.

For example, I took dance and exercise classes at night and I had a great group of friends that I enjoyed going out with on the weekends. Enjoying all of these other things in my life significantly decreased the stress I felt over school and provided me with outlets to alleviate that stress.

You need your own ways to express yourself that bring you joy and release. Partake in activities in which you aren't aiming to be the best or caring too much about a final product. You simply want to use these activities to relieve your stress and give you a needed break from your busy work schedule.

Once you have some outlets to relieve your stress, you should make sure that you schedule them into your life. For example, at the beginning of the week, make plans to go out with your friends on both Friday and Saturday nights. This will give you something to look forward to during the week and, when Friday rolls around, you'll be happy to have a much-needed and much-deserved break from your work.

Don't forget about scheduling in outlets for pleasure. They're important in order to keep you a happy, sane, student.

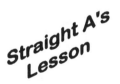

Make sure you have outlets in your life that are both fun and stress-relieving. Whether it's going out with your friends, exercising, or writing in a journal, make sure you take part in activities that take your mind off your busy school life.

Compete Only With Yourself

Compete only with yourself! You've probably heard that line before (perhaps you learned it for the first time in kindergarten). However, I do think it's a good message for the last chapter of this book.

It actually relates back to the beginning of this book. In Chapter One, we discussed the importance of setting goals. Now let's put a little spin on what I said earlier. Success is really a personal standard. It's about setting your own goals, doing everything you can to achieve them, and finally, reaching them. There is no objective standard out there to judge whether you have succeeded or not; success is reflective of what you set out to do in the first place.

If you view success as a personal standard, you'll soon realize that the only grades you should concern yourself with in each of your classes are your own. It really doesn't matter how well the person next to you did on the exam, it only matters how well you did in relation to the goal that you set for yourself.

Adopting this attitude will yield three important results:

1. **You'll excel for yourself:** When you aren't concerned about other's grades and you just concentrate on your own, you'll start achieving for your own benefit. You can always upgrade your own standards, but you might not be as motivated if you're setting your standards in relation to others who don't have that same determination as you.

2. **You'll be less stressed out:** If you judge your success according only to the goals you set for yourself, you'll likely be focused and calm. Why? Well for starters, you won't be caught up in the competitive rat race. Not worrying how other people are doing will save you from useless anxiety and leave you focused on your own goals and aspirations.

3. **You'll be a more likable classmate:** Choosing to compete only with yourself will mean that, for you, success won't depend on doing better than anyone else. If you view your classmates as competition, you'll carry a hostile attitude towards them. Competing only with yourself will leave you free to make friends and help people out whenever you have the time.

Don't bother to look over your shoulder to see how other people in your class did on an essay or exam. When you're applying to jobs or graduate programs, no one will be looking at the person next to you. You'll be the focus of their attention. Decide right away to concentrate on your own achievements and avoid comparing your accomplishments to those of your classmates' or friends'.

Straight A's Lesson

If you realize that success is a personal standard, you'll start to compete only with yourself. In the end, this attitude will push you to peak performance, decrease your level of stress, and make you a friendlier person to be around.

Commonly Asked Questions

Question: I love to get involved in extracurricular activities, but I find that I never have a chance to do my schoolwork because I'm too busy. I know getting involved in school is important, but am I doing too much?

Answer: It sounds like you are doing too much. Getting involved in extracurricular activities is voluntary. It's not the same as taking on a part-time job to support yourself. When these extracurricular activities become too time consuming for you, you want to give them less priority.

It's a good idea to get involved in extracurricular activities. It will make you a more interesting person and will give you a lot of things to record on your resume. As soon as your grades start to suffer because of your involvement, however, cut down on your activities.

If you can handle the juggling act of school and extracurricular activities – great! If not, you can still get involved in some activities - just don't get *as* involved.

Summary

I hope that this chapter gave you a good sense that it's entirely possible to have a life and at the same time, aim for school success. Work towards a balanced life while you're in school. It'll help you achieve your goals and will also help you develop into a well-rounded individual, full of energy and enthusiasm.

I've shown you that marks aren't everything in university. You've got to make friends, participate in extracurricular activities, and also find yourself challenging summer jobs. Also, I've emphasized the importance of taking care of yourself at university by eating well, exercising regularly, and ensuring you get a good night's sleep. Finally, you've got to try to remain calm in school by putting things into perspective. Do this by realizing there are a lot of second chances. Also, create outlets to relieve your stress and decide to compete only with yourself. If you stick to everything I have suggested, you should be able to succeed in school, and at the same time, have a memorable experience.

APPENDIX

WEBSITES FOR STUDENTS

APARTMENTS IN CANADA

http://www.carol.ca (Canadian apartments for rent online)
http://www.rent.net

APARTMENTS IN THE UNITED STATES

http://www.apartmentguide.com
http://www.apartments.com
http://www.apartmentsforrent.com
http://www.apartmentworld.com
http://www.homestore.com
http://www.rent.net

ESSAY WRITING SITES

Accepted.com

http://www.accepted.com

This website is for anyone applying for admission to medical school, law school, business school, or any other graduate programs. Learn how to write essays that will help get you into these programs.

The Columbia Guide to Online Style

http://www.cas.usf.edu/english/walker/mla.html

An easy to use guide to MLA (Modern Language Association)-Style Citations of Electronic Sources (Internet Sources).

Essay Punch

http://www.essaypunch.com

This website takes users through the steps of writing a short essay. Step-by-step, users are prompted to go through the essay writing process that includes pre-writing, writing, organizing, editing, and rewriting.

Essay Writing for Students in Politics and Social Sciences

http://www.pol.adfa.edu.au/resources/essay_writing/part_3.html

Essay Writing Guide

http://www.arts.monash.edu.au/history/essaywri/essaywri.htm

How to Organize a Research Paper and Document it with MLA Citations

http://www.geocities.com/Athens/oracle/4184

This website provides important information about organizing a research paper. Most importantly, it can help you document sources in the bibliographic format recommended by the Modern Language Association (MLA). Made for beginning writers, it is straightforward and easy to use.

MLA Bibliographic Citation Guide

http://www.sccd.ctc.edu/~library/mlacite.html

This website provides the correct citation form for a variety of materials such as books, reference sources, periodical articles, full text articles from electronic databases, government publications, and World Wide Web resources.

Nelson Political Science – Essay Writing Reference Resource

http://www.polisci.nelson.com/reference.html

This website links to useful reference resources for essay writing, including essay writing guidelines, citation guides, and on-line dictionaries and grammar aids.

Paradigm Online Writing Assistant

http://www.powa.org

This website contains tips on writing the following types of essays: informal, thesis/support, argumentative, exploratory. It also provides information on organizing, revising, editing, and documenting sources in your essay.

Plagiary and the Art of Skillful Citation

http://condor.bcm.tmc.edu/Micro-Immuno/courses/igr/homeric.html

If you want to make sure you're not doing anything illegal when you're writing a research paper, you might want to take a look at the article posted on this website, "How to Cite Skillfully and Avoid Plagiarizing".

Research & Writing for High School and College Students

http://www.ipl.org/teen/aplus

This website provides a step-by-step guide to researching and writing a paper. It can help you learn about and perform information searches in cyberspace and in your library. In addition, it contains important links to other online resources for research and writing.

Research Paper

http://www.researchpaper.com

Among other things, this website contains an idea directory that includes over four thousand topics. It also contains a writing center with writing tips and technique guidelines.

A Student's Guide to Research with the World Wide Web

http://www.slu.edu/departments/english/research

This is a tutorial guide to conducting research on the Internet. It aims to help you explore World Wide Web resources and to give you strategies for evaluating the usefulness of websites.

EXAMS: WRITING AND PREPARATION

Answering Essay Questions on Exams

http://www.utexas.edu/student/lsc/handouts/1446.html
http://www.cl.uh.edu/ssc/sca/lss/keyword.htm
http://www.utexas.edu/student/lsc/handouts/1419.html

Anticipating Test Content

http://www.iss.stthomas.edu/studyguides/tstprp2.htm

Bloom's Hierarchy of Test Questions

http://quarles.unbc.ca/lsc/bloom.html

Index of Learning Styles Questionnaire

http://www2.ncsu.edu/unity/lockers/users/f/felder/public/ILSdir/ilsweb.html

After you answer 44 quick questions you can submit your results to get a summary of your learning style.

Learning Styles

http://snow.utoronto.ca/Learn2/mod3/miinventory.html

Free Education on the Internet

http://www.free-ed.net

Free online courses, tutorials, and study guides.

How to Keep Calm During Tests

http://www.cl.uh.edu/ssc/sca/lss/calmtest.htm
http://www.utexas.edu/student/lsc/handouts/1305.html

How to Survive Exam Week

http://www.utexas.edu/student/lsc/handouts/1427.html

Learning from Your Returned Exam

http://www.sdc.uwo.ca/learning/mcreturn.html

Multiple Choice Exams

http://www.sdc.uwo.ca/learning/mcintro.html
http://www.utexas.edu/student/lsc/handouts/1444.html
http://quarles.unbc.ca/lsc/jtmulcho.html
http://128.32.89.153/CalRen/TestsObjective.html
http://www.coun.uvic.ca/learn/program/hndouts/multicho.html

Organizing for Tests

http://www.iss.stthomas.edu/studyguides/tstprp6.htm

Problem-Solving Tests

http://www.utexas.edu/student/lsc/handouts/1443.html

Review Tools for Tests

http://www.iss.stthomas.edu/studyguides/tstprp5.htm

Study Guides and Strategies

http://www.iss.stthomas.edu/studyguides

This website contains tips on preparing to learn, participating in classrooms, studying, reading skills, preparing for tests, taking tests, writing skills, and writing essays.

Study Skills

http://www.tsd.jcu.edu.au/netshare/learn/studskls/online.html

Information on organizing yourself, learning, attending lectures and tutorials, and writing essays and exams.

Tips on Test-Taking

http://depthome.brooklyn.cuny.edu/career/HOWTEST.HTM

Test Anxiety – How to Reduce and Manage It

http://www.iss.stthomas.edu/studyguides/tstprp8.htm
http://www.rhbnc.ac.uk/~uhye099/exams.html
http://www.counsel.wsu.edu/csweb/howto.htm
http://www.ksu.edu/ucs/strestst.html
http://www.sdc.uwo.ca/learning/mcanx.html
http://www.ksu.edu/ucs/stresgen.html

GENERAL RESOURCES

Graduate Student Resources Page

http://www-personal.umich.edu/~danhorn/graduate.html

Online Dictionary

http://www.dictionary.com

Online Thesaurus

http://www.thesaurus.com

Student Sites

http://www.essay.com
http://www.student.com
http://www.studentmkt.com
http://www.studentadvantage.com

GRAMMAR RESOURCES

ABCheckers

http://webnz.com/checkers

This is an English language consulting company that was set up in 1995 by a group of New Zealand teachers. The aim is to help people improve their English skills. For example, one useful thing you can do is to send your essays to them over the Internet to be corrected for a fee.

The American Heritage® Book of English Usage

http://www.bartleby.com/64

This website contains a guide to contemporary English that may help your writing style and answer any questions you have regarding English grammar.

The English Institute's Grammar Book

http://62.6.162.42/intro.html

This website includes simple lessons in grammar that might teach you a thing or two about nouns, pronouns, indefinite articles, etc.

HEALTH

"Dr. Steve" on Substance Abuse

http://www.DrSteve.org

Steve Adelman, M.D., claims to be an authority on substance use, substance abuse, addiction and recovery. His, "goal is to help people figure out where to draw the line in order to regain a healthy balance in their lives".

Health on the Net Foundation (HON)

http://www.hon.ch

You can search this site for healthcare websites, hospitals and support.

Mediconsult

http://www.mediconsult.com

This virtual medical center provides lots of information on a wide range of medical conditions.

Medscout: Medical Reference Information

http://www.medscout.com

Wellness Center

http://tigger.stthomas.edu/well

Wellness and drug education at the University of St. Thomas

JOBS IN CANADA

http://www.studentjobs.com
http://www.workpolis.ca
http://www.monster.ca
http://www.careerclick.com

JOBS IN THE UNITED STATES

http://www.monster.com
http://www.ajb.dni.us
http://www.jobtrak.com
http://www.jobbankusa.com
http://www.jobweb.org
http://www.collegegrad.com
http://www.job-hunt.org
http://www.jobdirect.com

SCHOLARSHIPS AND FINANCIAL AID FOR COLLEGE/UNIVERSITY

Best College Scholarships

http://rusty.hypermart.net/college.htm

Here you'll find lists to many private scholarships.

Cashe

http://www.mgslp.state.mt.us/cashe~1.html

Cashe (College Aid Source for Higher Education) is a respected source of financial aid resources for college. It also provides a free scholarship search program.

College Scholarships

http://www.myfreeoffice.com/underfoot/college.html

At this website 10 scholarship search engines are brought together.

College-Scholarships

http://www.college-scholarships.com

This site contains information about college and universities throughout the U.S. It also provides free college scholarship and financial aid searches.

The Collegiate Websource – Go College

http://www.gocollege.com

It's thought to be the largest scholarship database available.

EDU

http://www.usnews.com/usnews/edu/dollars/scholar/search.htm

Find a scholarship by using this "U.S. World and News" engine that divides scholarships into six categories: ethnic, athletic, art, corporate, organizational, and military.

Embark

http://www.embark.com

Brings together various educational financial resources.

Expan

http://www.collegeboard.org/fundfinder/html/ssrchtop.html

This is the College Board's Free Scholarship Search Program. "Here you can locate scholarships, loans, internships, and other financial aid programs from non-college sources that match your education level, talents, and background". It contains a database of 2000 undergrad scholarships, internships, and loan programs.

FASTWEB

http://www.fastweb.com

This is a free scholarship search database containing 400,000 scholarships.

Financial Aid Website Index

http://www.finaid.org

Go to this website to find out about loans, scholarships, and grants for college/university.

24x7 Free College Scholarships Directory

http://www.scholarships-free-colleges-grants-minorities.com

Free-Scholarships-and-Financial Aid

http://www.free-scholarships-and-financial-aid.com

Go to this website to discover scholarships and financial aid programs for which you may qualify.

FRESCH

http://www.freschinfo.com/index.phtml

This website contains a database of over 2000 organizations and foundations that offer scholarships that represent about 169,000 awards.

International Student

http://www.internationalstudent.com

If you are an international student who wants to attend a university in the U.S., then this website can help you find information and link you to other sites with information about scholarships for international students.

Mach 25 – "Breaking the Tuition Barrier"

http://www.collegenet.com/mach25

The College Net scholarship search includes 600,000 awards totaling over $1.6 billion.

Nationally Coveted Scholarships

http://www.scholarships.kachinatech.com/scholarships/scholars.html

"Highly competitive and prestigious awards for college, graduate school, and postgraduate study".

Peterson's College Quest

http://www.collegequest.com

Explore colleges and financial aid options at this site.

The Scholarship Page

http://4a2z.4anything.com/home

At this website you can search for scholarships by keyword or browse.

Scholarships Canada

http://www.scholarshipscanada.com

Free scholarship database offering customizable searches and tips on how to apply.

SRN Express

http://www.rams.com/srn

SRN Express (Scholarship Research Network Express) is a search engine and database containing private scholarships. It also has information about student loan forgiveness programs for those who've graduated from college and need alternative ways for repaying debt.

Tuitions, Loans, Grants, and Jobs on College Campuses

http://www.mo.nea.org/college/tuition.htm

Apply electronically for many financial services.

Win Scholarships

http://www.winscholarships.com

Learn how to win scholarships and receive financial aid at this website.

INDEX

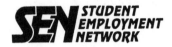
SEN STUDENT EMPLOYMENT NETWORK

THREE GREAT PUBLICATIONS!

Ten Ways To Straight A's

A brand new book that offers valuable insight into the secrets of succeeding in school and beyond. Learn how to get your mind set on school success, how to write effective essays, survive exam time, and much more! The author, an average student herself at the beginning, has developed a formula that has helped her achieve school success. Now, she is a student at Harvard Law School!

**188 pages
ISBN 1-896324-36-3
$19.95**

The Canada Student Employment Guide (2001 Edition)

Now fully updated and expanded! This year the book contains almost 1,000 employer profiles with contact info, academic fields and skills companies seek, and part time and summer employment information. New this year is a section on co-op and internship opportunities! This book is the most valuable employment reference guide for students!

**720 pages
ISBN 1-896324-34-7
$26.95**

The Canadian Job Directory (Year 2000/2001 Edition)

A popular resource for both adults and students that contains hundreds of profiles on every imaginable source of employment including: Firms and Organizations; Recruiters; Trade Assoc.; Career Resources on the Internet; and Human Resource Canada Centres. It is an essential job seeker's guide!

**462 pages
ISBN 1-896324-30-4
$ 24.95**

To Order

Please send me ____ copy(s) of *Ten Ways to Straight A's*

Please send me ____ copy(s) of *The Canada Student Employment Guide (2000 Ed.)*

Please send me ____ copy(s) of *The Canadian Job Directory (2000/2001 Ed.)*

Enclosed is a cheque/money order for $ _____ (payable to SEN)

Please add $6.00 Shipping plus 7% GST to all orders (HST & QST where applicable).

Name: _____

Address: _____ City: _____

Prov: _____ Postal Code: _____ Tel: _____

**Student Employment Network
117 Gerrard Street East, Suite 1002, Toronto, ON, M5B 2L4
Tel: (416) 971-5090   Fax: (416) 977-3782
Internet: www.studentjobs.com   E-mail: sen@studentjobs.com**

Discounts are available for larger orders. Contact the publisher above for more information.